Pharmaceutical policy in China:
challenges and opportunities for reform

Pharmaceutical policy in China: challenges and opportunities for reform

Elias Mossialos, Yanfeng Ge, Jia Hu and Liejun Wang

London School of Economics and Political Science
and
Development Research Center of the State Council of China

Keywords
DRUG AND NARCOTIC CONTROL
PHARMACEUTICAL PREPARATIONS
DRUG COSTS
DRUG INDUSTRY
HEALTH CARE REFORM
HEALTH POLICY
CHINA

Address requests about publications to: Publications, WHO Regional Office for Europe, UN City, Marmorvej 51, DK-2100 Copenhagen Ø, Denmark.

Alternatively, complete an online request form for documentation, health information, or for permission to quote or translate, on the Regional Office web site (www.euro.who.int/pubrequest).

ISBN 978 92 890 5039 5

Printed in the United Kingdom
Copy editing by Jane Ward
Design by Sarah Moncrieff

Contents

Acknowledgements

We would like to graciously thank Bo Wang and the Shanghai Medical Innovation Foundation for their support of this project.

We would like to thank the Organisation of Economic Co-operation and Development, World Health Organization, Boston Consulting Group, IMS Health, Kieger, McKinsey, the *Journal of the American Medical Association* and *Therapeutic Innovation & Regulatory Science* for allowing us to reuse figures found in their reports and publications in this report.

We would like thank the following section contributors for their assistance in research and drafting: Wrik Ghosh (Chapter 12), Raymond Kennedy (Chapter 14), Tyler Law (Chapters 5, 6 and 8), Austin Le (Chapters 4 and 9) and Angela Yu (Chapter 10).

Finally, we would like to thank Jeffrey Moe, Shenglan Tang and Di Dong from Duke Kunshan University for reviewing the report and the collaboration with the Asia Pacific Observatory on Health Systems and Policies in facilitating their review.

All remaining errors are those of the authors.

List of abbreviations

AIDS	Acquired immunodeficiency syndrome
API	Active Pharmaceutical Ingredient
BRICS	Brazil, Russia, India, China and South Africa
CDE	Center for Drug Evaluation
CER	Comparative effectiveness research
CFDA	China Food and Drug Administration
CHC	Community health centre
EDL	Essential Drug List
EU	European Union
GDP	Gross domestic product
GMP	Good Manufacturing Practice
HIV	Human immunodeficiency virus
HTA	Health technology assessment
IRP	Internal reference pricing
NCD	Noncommunicable disease
NCMS	New Cooperative Medical Scheme
NDA	New drug application
NDRC	National Development and Reform Commission
NHFPC	National Health and Family Planning Commission
NRDL	National Reimbursement Drug List
OECD	Organisation of Economic Co-operation and Development
OOP	Out of pocket
OTC	Over the counter
R&D	Research and development
TCM	Traditional Chinese medicine
THC	Township health centre
THE	Total health expenditure
TPE	Total pharmaceutical expenditure
UEBMI	Urban Employee Basic Medical Insurance
URBMI	Urban Resident Basic Medical Insurance
US FDA	United States Food and Drug Administration
WHO	World Health Organization
ZMU	Zero mark-up

List of tables, figures and boxes

Tables

Figures

Boxes

1. Introduction and report overview

1.1 Objectives and challenges of pharmaceutical policy

Pharmaceuticals make a significant contribution to the health and well-being of a population and government policy regarding pharmaceuticals exerts a significant effect on the state of the pharmaceutical market. Governments generally have several objectives when developing pharmaceutical policy. For example, the World Health Organization (WHO) suggests that a national pharmaceutical policy should adhere to three key principles (WHO, 2001):

- access: equitable availability and affordability of essential drugs;
- quality: ensuring all medicines are safe and efficacious; and
- rational use: promoting therapeutically sound and cost-effective use of medications for health providers and patients.

Broadly speaking, pharmaceutical policy objectives can be divided into two overarching categories: health policy objectives and industrial policy objectives. Health policy objectives include quality, macroeconomic efficiency, microeconomic efficiency and health equity. Quality refers to having a supply of safe and efficacious medications. Macroeconomic efficiency relates to spending on pharmaceuticals and how that fits into overall health care and government expenditures. While cost-containment is not necessarily an objective in and of itself, it is a consideration in balancing conflicting spending demands. Microeconomic efficiency refers to the cost-effective allocation of resources and takes into account factors such as specific drug pricing and needs-based allocation. Finally, most governments prioritize equity, which means equal access based on need rather than income.

A dimension of complexity is added when industrial policy is an objective, as there is often a tension between health policy goals and industrial policy goals. Examples of industrial policy objectives include supporting the pharmaceutical industry though encouraging research and development (R&D), ensuring strong employment in the pharmaceutical sector and creating an export-oriented industry. Fostering R&D generally involves giving patent protection to innovative products, which gives firms a monopoly and the ability to charge higher prices on their products. This directly clashes with many of the health policy objectives described above. Balancing policies such that true innovation is appropriately rewarded and new drugs are developed while keeping prices as affordable as possible is challenging.

The complexity of the pharmaceutical market makes it unique in the extent to which it is not a "perfect market" (Abel-Smith & Grandjeat, 1978; Dukes et al., 2003; Jacobzone, 2000). From a supply-side perspective, problems arise through the importance of patent protection; the complexity and length of regulatory approval; the importance of ensuring quality, because patients lack the ability to discern "good" products from "bad"; and brand loyalty. From a demand-side perspective, there is a many tiered consumer structure in which physicians prescribe, pharmacists dispense (or in the case of China, hospitals dispense), patients consume and payment can be made by public or private insurers or by the patients themselves. The market is generally characterized by information asymmetry (i.e. patients do not know which drugs they need; patients and physicians do not know which drugs are necessarily safe, high quality and efficacious) and externalities (i.e. ineffective treatment in one group can lead to negative health outcomes in another, particularly when it comes to infectious diseases). Consequently, strong regulations and effective policies are particularly important in the pharmaceutical environment.

Whatever a country's objectives, it is crucial to monitor any policy changes using high-quality data. Pharmaceutical policies can often have unintended consequences that spill over into other areas of the health care system. It is only through careful evaluation that a government can ensure that its policies are in line with overall objectives. Some of the key aspects of pharmaceutical policy and how they tie into overall objectives are explored below.

1.1.1 Market authorization, drug approvals and drug quality

In order for pharmaceuticals to be used by patients, they must first receive market authorization and approval. Most countries have a specific agency responsible for both authorizations and quality: the Food and Drug Administration in the United States (US FDA), the European Medicines Agency in Europe and the Chinese Food and Drug Administration (CFDA) in China. The regulatory requirements behind drug approvals are complex and can take years to navigate as pharmaceuticals are very different from other consumer goods.

To be approved by a regulatory agency, a pharmaceutical must meet the three standards of safety, efficacy and quality. A fourth component, postmarketing surveillance, exists to ensure that drug effects that are not known during the relatively brief period of clinical testing can be detected when on the market. This is an important part of risk mitigation, since prior to approval it is impossible to know if a drug will be completely safe. In order for drugs to be demonstrably efficacious, high-quality clinical data in the form of randomized clinical trials is required. Ideally, such testing would be carried out against the best currently available treatments, as this would indicate which drugs were truly clinically superior compared with those already available.

This comparative effectiveness research (CER) can be extremely helpful in guiding the approvals and pricing and reimbursement process. Health technology assessment (HTA) is a variant of CER that also incorporates economic factors in addition to clinical effectiveness. In mature markets, this is often the final hurdle before drugs gain marketing approval or reimbursement values are set. Unfortunately, new drugs are often only compared with placebos and can gain approval without rigorous CER. While more regulatory agencies are incorporating CER and HTA into their approval process, there is still a long way to go for many jurisdictions, including China.

From an approvals perspective, another important goal is to ensure that new medications are approved in a timely fashion for both novel patent drugs that yield clinical benefit and generic drugs for products that are coming off-patent and will yield cost savings. This requires that the approvals agency has sufficient regulatory capacity. In the past, the US FDA has had difficulties, with limited capacity leading to delays in drug approvals. This led to legislation that allowed fees to be levied from industry to increase capacity, which was ultimately successful at reducing delays in approvals (PhRMA, 2015). Another way for new drugs of significant importance to receive timely approval is to create a channel for priority reviews or forms of review (breakthrough, fast track or accelerated approvals) that are allowed to use surrogate clinical end-points rather than final trial data.

Ensuring drug quality is another important role of the regulatory agencies and requires both strong regulations for Good Manufacturing Practice (GMP) and effective inspection capacity. An effective postmarketing surveillance system to identify adverse effects once drugs leave the factory is also essential. Specifically for generic medications, mandating that they be tested against the right reference drug (i.e. off-patent originator) is necessary. In the United States, these reference drugs have been codified into the US FDA's Orange Book. Many jurisdictions, including China, do not have such a reference for comparison of off-patent originators. This opens the possibility for potential quality concerns.

1.1.2 Pricing and reimbursement

The goal of pricing and reimbursement policy is not cost-containment per se but rather to ensure that prices and reimbursement levels reflect a drug's actual value and that a degree of affordability is maintained. Supply-side measures seek to directly target the prices of pharmaceutical products and include measures such as direct price controls, external reference pricing (international reference pricing), tendering and the use of HTA. Reimbursement policies include internal reference pricing (IRP) and tiered reimbursement.

Direct price controls, which include price setting, price ceilings and price cuts, are widely used throughout the European Union (EU) but less so in the United States, which has little in the way of direct pricing regulation. In general, European governments tend to be larger, single purchaser markets, which are, therefore, more capable of enforcing direct controls. The United States uses indirect price controls and market competition because of the large number of health insurers. While such price controls lead to short-term decreases in prices, in the medium to long-term they tend to be compensated for by volume increases (Carone, Schwierz & Xavier, 2012). In general, overall increases in pharmaceutical spending are driven by volume increases or the introduction of new pharmaceuticals in spite of direct price regulation (Mossialos, Mrazek & Walley, 2004). External reference pricing (international reference pricing) is another commonly used policy, which takes the form of setting a maximum price per standardized unit based on prices in other countries. In reality, external reference pricing is technically challenging as acquiring actual drug prices is very difficult since pharmaceutical companies definitely prefer to keep such data confidential. Tendering, in which manufacturers make competitive blinded bids for contracts to provide pharmaceuticals for a particular insurer, region or institution, has been effective at obtaining significant cost savings. Evidence from the Netherlands and Germany has demonstrated drastic reductions in prices, in the order of 80–90% (Kanavos, Seeley & Vandoros, 2009). The long-term effects on market dynamics, competition and supply sustainability are not clear. Finally, tenders tend to be on the basis of price alone, a factor that assumes an identical product in which quality is not of concern.

HTA can be very useful for the pricing of new medications. It is being used increasingly throughout the EU, with the United Kingdom's National Institute for Health and Care Excellence one of the world's HTA leaders. HTA assesses the additional value of a medicine relative to existing alternatives and takes into account both clinical effectiveness and cost. It can be used for market authorization, pricing or reimbursement. While HTA is very appealing from its ability to combine true clinical value with cost, it can be technically challenging to perform.

IRP is a commonly used reimbursement policy in which maximum prices for reimbursement are set. For generics, this maximum price is often defined as a percentage of the off-patent originator's price. A very important element of IRP is how large the reference cluster is: for identical molecules (i.e. all types of atorvastatin, a cholesterol-lowering drug of the statin class), for molecules of the same class (i.e. for all statins) or for molecules with similar therapeutic effect (i.e. for all cholesterol-lowering drugs, including statins, fibrates and others). Defining what is "therapeutically interchangeable" is one of the most important aspects of IRP and can be a point of significant contention. An advantage of IRP is that it makes patients and physicians more price sensitive, particularly for drugs considered to be identical (i.e. off-patent originators versus generics). For example, patients must pay for the difference between actual and reference price if they choose to use a higher-priced medication.

Tiered reimbursement, where products are differentially reimbursed on the basis of effectiveness, can be another useful means of signalling value to providers and patients. This is similar to value-based user charges, where the patient co-payment increases with decreasing clinical value (Thomson, Schang & Chernew, 2013). Using either of these measures requires CER to inform the value and subsequent reimbursement structure of various products.

1.1.3 Influencing physicians, pharmacists and the supply chain

Physicians are key players in the pharmaceutical market since they, and not patients, tend to be the key drivers of demand. Good prescribing includes choosing a medication that is clinically appropriate for the patient in a way that maximizes effectiveness, minimizes harm from side-effects and is as cost-effective as possible (Barber, 1995).

Various policies are capable of enhancing prescribing effectiveness. These include monitoring prescribing quality, including a feedback mechanism; the use of clinical practice guidelines; direct educational programmes; and academic detailing. Medical training also plays a foundational role in teaching effective clinical prescribing. Most physician-directed interventions can also be linked to financial incentives, either positive or negative, to guide behaviour.

Even if physicians are prescribing the most clinically effective medications, they might not necessarily be prescribing the cheapest ones. This is particularly the case when it comes to medications for which generic alternatives are available. Consequently, prescription by international nonproprietary name is one important way in which to promote the use of generics and thereby lower costs. Another cost-containment measure is the use of prescription budgets, in which penalties can be triggered when prescribing by individual physicians, or groups of physicians, exceeds a certain dollar amount.

One of the most important interventions at the pharmacy level is the use of generic substitution, which is the right of a pharmacist to replace a medication (e.g. an expensive off-patent originator) with another that has the identical active ingredient (a cheap generic). In general, replacing off-patent originators with generic medications can yield significant cost savings without any adverse health effects, assuming that the two products are indeed identical. One study estimated the total savings in the EU to be €43 billion, or about 33% of public total pharmaceutical expenditure (TPE) with total generic substitution (Carone, Schwierz & Xavier, 2012).

Regulation of how distributors and pharmacists are paid is also important. Wholesalers and pharmacists are given large discounts by drug manufacturers to sell their products, particularly in the case of generic medications. These can be as much as 70% of the price of the drug itself (Kanavos & Taylor, 2007). Limiting the amount of these discounts can yield significant cost savings. Furthermore, if pharmacy remuneration is based on the percentage of drug price, this will incentivize the dispensing of more-expensive medications. Consequently, having either fixed prescribing fees or even regressive fees (in which pharmacists make more when cheaper medications are prescribed) is efficient.

1.1.4 Linking pharmaceutical policies with health policy objectives

Quality, the first of the health policy objectives, is very much linked with the market authorization and the quality regulatory environment. Consequently, it is important to have strong policies and a regulator with sufficient capacity and oversight. That being said, the way in which drugs are priced and reimbursed can also affect quality: Specifically one of China's current problems is that tendering does not take drug quality very seriously, which creates a market incentive to prioritize lower cost at the expense of quality. Allowing manufacturers to participate in tendering only after meeting quality criteria could be a way of improving the quality of tendered drugs, and this approach has been used in Germany and Australia.

Macroeconomic efficiency is a challenge in China as pharmaceutical expenditure makes up nearly 40% of total health expenditure (THE), a combination of both relatively high prices and excessive amounts of prescribing. Such a high level of spending in some senses crowds out allocation to other areas of health care, such as spending on physicians and hospitals. Ironically, as a significant proportion of health provider revenue is derived from drug sales, there is an incentive to prescribe more medications, feeding a vicious cycle of pharmaceutical overspending. Reforms to improve microeconomic efficiency are needed to address this macroeconomic problem.

Many policies can influence microeconomic efficiency. From a patient perspective, reimbursement policies such as IRP and tiered reimbursement can lead to more rational use of medicines. Policies that encourage physician overprescribing (such as being allowed to earn profits from drug sales, or salaries that are too low) will undermine efficiency. From a pharmacist and distribution perspective, microeconomic efficiency can be promoted through generic substitution and reducing fragmentation. Ultimately, the goal of microeconomic efficiency – cost-effective allocation of pharmaceuticals based on need – requires alignment of a number of policies.

Ensuring equity is an important goal in and of itself and in maintaining microeconomic efficiency. If access to drugs is based on ability to pay rather than need, then those with high need and low means will have difficulties accessing treatment. This would be an inefficient allocation of resources. Reimbursement policies that minimize out-of-pocket (OOP) payments and are equal regardless of income level are essential for equity.

It is clear that these four health policy objectives are closely related. Promoting microeconomic efficiency means ensuring there is equity; microeconomic efficiency is required for macroeconomic efficiency; and macroeconomic efficiency and quality are necessary for overall health objectives to be met.

1.1.5 Industrial policy and intellectual property

Conceptually, an effective pharmaceutical industry is necessary for any country to have drugs to use in its health system in the first place. However, balancing the desire for innovation (through patent protection) and for access to affordable medications can be difficult. New drugs are protected through an extensive network of product and process patents along with data exclusivity (protection of safety and efficacy data on drugs without which generic medications cannot seek approval). The rationale for such protection is in order to stimulate the innovation and investment necessary – in the order of hundreds of millions of dollars – to develop new medications. Against this, the monopoly prices that companies are able to charge can be excessive and significantly impede access, particularly for the less well-off.

For some conditions for which there are very few patients (orphan diseases), regular patent protection has been insufficient to promote drug development. As a result, various regulations such as the Orphan Drug Act in the United States and Orphan Designation under the European Medicines Agency have increased the degree of protection and marketing exclusivity these drugs have. These regulations have been successful in increasing the number of drugs developed to treat orphan diseases. On the other end of the spectrum, regulations have also been put in place to allow for rapid introduction of generics. Many countries have implemented Bolar provisions, which allow for research comparing generic drugs with originators to be carried out during the patent protection period. This enables generics to enter the market as soon as patents expire. The Hatch–Waxman Act in the United States also grants a period of marketing exclusivity to the first generic drug on the market, which encourages rapid entry of generic manufacturers. Striking the right balance between too much and too little protection can be one of the most challenging tasks regulators must face.

China faces a number of challenges from an industrial policy and intellectual property standpoint. It has lagged in the production of both high-quality generic drugs and in promoting pharmaceutical R&D. The latter is in part caused by problems with a sometimes weak intellectual property regime. The pharmaceutical market is also plagued with significant fragmentation, characterized by a multitude of small manufacturers incapable of maintaining quality standards or innovating. Local protectionism of weak firms is a key driver of this landscape. All-in-all, a coherent industrial policy that takes into account objectives such as innovation and the production of affordable, quality generics would be quite helpful but does not currently exist.

1.2 Report overview

China's pharmaceutical environment, characterized by fragmented regulation and perverse market incentives, faces many challenges including problems with drug quality, access and affordability; irrational medicine use; and high drug prices. However, as the second world's largest market by value, there are many opportunities to create a pharmaceutical industry capable of providing affordable quality medicines for its people and the world. This report provides a comprehensive and current overview of pharmaceutical policy in China. Each chapter covers a topic important to China's pharmaceutical environment and is briefly described below:

Chapter 2: *Introduction to Chinese health care reform and pharmaceutical policy.* This chapter provides historical context to China's health care system. China rapidly transitioned from a government-administered system to a market-oriented one in the 1980s. This was accompanied by large declines in government spending and commensurate increases in private spending. One of the most perverse policies was the 15% mark-up, which allowed hospitals and doctors make a profit from drug sales. As government funding dwindled, health care providers became reliant on drug revenues to survive. Overprescribing and challenges with access and affordability ensued. In 2009, the government launched sweeping reforms aimed at overhauling the health care system. Five priority areas were identified, including broadening health insurance, strengthening the public health system, improving primary care, reforming public hospitals and lastly reforming China's pharmaceutical system and introducing the Essential Drug List (EDL). While some successes have been achieved, China has a long way to go before its health care reforms can realize its goals of affordable access to health care for all.

Chapter 3: *Regulatory structure and drug approval.* China has a highly fragmented regulatory structure for health care and has many problems with its drug approval process. Responsibility for pharmaceutical policy falls across many different ministries at the central level while provincial agencies exert considerable influence in policy formulation and implementation. Unfortunately, there is no national pharmaceutical strategy that coordinates policy development, which results in fragmented decision-making. The CFDA is the ministry responsible for new drug approvals and monitoring drug quality. Significant understaffing and an irrational drug approval process that does not prioritize important or innovative drugs has led to a large backlog in new drug applications (NDAs) and insufficient monitoring of drug quality. Since 2014, there have been many new policy announcements aimed at addressing some of these regulatory challenges.

Chapter 4: *Key health issues: ageing, urbanization and noncommunicable diseases.* Over the past several decades, health outcomes in China have dramatically improved but moving forward there will be many difficult health challenges to contend with. China is undergoing a significant epidemiological transition as noncommunicable diseases (NCDs) are replacing infectious diseases as the main causes of mortality and morbidity. China has an ageing population, increasingly unhealthy lifestyle habits from rapid urbanization and some of the highest smoking rates in the world. This has led to a rapid increase in rates of NCDs such as diabetes, cardiovascular diseases and cancer. Dealing with the rise of these NCDs will require a coordinated health system response that involves public health and primary care, strong regulations and a pharmaceutical system able to deliver quality, affordable medicines for these conditions.

Chapter 5: *Trends in health care and pharmaceutical spending.* China is spending an increasing amount on health care, with double-digit gains that has outpaced gross domestic product (GDP) growth. In spite of gains in health care spending, China still spends far less than countries of the Organisation of Economic Co-operation and Development (OECD) as a percentage of GDP. Furthermore, there is significant geographical variation in spending and OOP expenditure remains high. China spends a much higher proportion of its health care expenditure on drugs than most other countries. Growth in drug spending has been very high but increases are projected to decline in the coming years. Most of this spending occurs in hospitals rather than pharmacies, which is also different from most countries. China's drug market is dominated by off-patent drugs by value, but in the future the size of both the patent drug market and the EDL market is set to increase.

Chapter 6: *Affordability and accessibility of pharmaceuticals.* Despite significant increases in government investment in health care, there is still a perception that health care is expensive. The depth of insurance coverage is still very shallow, with high co-payments and low ceilings, particularly for the New Cooperative Medical Scheme (NCMS) and the Urban Resident Basic Medical Insurance (URBMI) system. Studies on the affordability of medicines demonstrate that, while generic medications were generally appropriately priced, off-patent originators were much higher in price. Surveys also demonstrate that accessibility for many medicines is challenging. OOP spending still accounts for a large share of total health spending and even disposable income, particularly for rural Chinese. There is much to be done in terms of health insurance, drug pricing and drug reimbursement in order to improve affordability and access.

Chapter 7: *Pharmaceutical pricing and reimbursement.* Pricing and reimbursement has been one of the most dynamic policy areas in recent years. Direct price controls, which had been used for decades, were eliminated in summer 2015. The 15% mark-up, which has incentivized irrational prescribing, is also gradually being phased out through the zero mark-up (ZMU) policy. Tendering is China's strongest supply-side pricing strategy, but there has been an overreliance on price that has compromised drug quality. Furthermore, local protectionism means that tenders will sometimes be awarded on the basis of patronage rather than merit. The government is planning on introducing reimbursement caps, a type of IRP, which could hypothetically guide rational prescribing and narrow the gap in price between locally made generics and off-patent originators. Unfortunately, there is a general lack of HTA or CER in any part of pharmaceutical decision-making. China has two main reimbursements lists, the EDL and the National Reimbursement Drug List (NRDL). The latter has not been updated since 2009, which means that most new drugs must be paid for by patients. China would do well to develop a more coherent national pricing and reimbursement strategy that pays heed to these issues.

Chapter 8: *Drug quality and supply chain.* Drug quality is a serious problem in China. A lack of bioequivalence testing and strong GMP standards, significant market fragmentation leading to thousands of manufacturers and understaffing at regulatory authorities all contribute to the problem. This has led to huge price differences between off-patent originators from multinational corporations and local generics and to difficulties with export. The distribution supply chain is also heavily fragmented and this has led to significant mark-ups from factory to patient. Recent policy changes have called for higher quality standards and increased CFDA capacity, both steps in the right direction. Increasing the capacity of the CFDA and promoting consolidation will also be crucial in improving China's pharmaceutical landscape.

Chapter 9: *Irrational prescribing.* Irrational prescribing is a serious problem in China, with rates of antibiotic and injection use far higher than recommended by international guidelines. This has been driven by the 15% mark-up policy and patients' expectations that these treatments were necessary. Over-prescribing has led to high rates of antimicrobial resistance and adverse drug events. There have also been problems with poor drug adherence and drug interactions. The government has implemented policies to encourage rational prescribing such as the ZMU policy and national antibiotic stewardship campaigns. China must continue to improve the quality of prescribing by promoting physician and patient education, providing incentives for good prescribing and using clinical support tools such as practice guidelines and electronic medical records.

Chapter 10: *Hospitals and pharmaceutical policy.* A weak primary care system means China relies heavily on its hospitals for the provision of both inpatient and outpatient services. Hospitals account for about 65% of THE as well as 70–80% of TPE. As hospitals are the main arbiters of care, health care reform is not possible without hospital reform. One of the most important yet most challenging reforms has been the introduction of ZMU in hospitals to remove the link between drug sales (which account for 40% of hospital revenues, four times greater than direct government subsidies) and general hospital revenues. At county hospitals where ZMU has been more widely implemented, revenues from drugs have decreased but unfortunately government subsidies and medical service fees have not made up for lost revenue. In order for ZMU to rationalize prescribing in China's huge hospital sector, comprehensive hospital payment reform that rewards quality care instead of overprescribing is needed.

Chapter 11: *Primary care and pharmaceutical policy.* A good primary care system has been shown to improve access, quality, preventive care and efficiency. Recognizing the weaknesses of China's primary care system, the government made primary care reform one of the five pillars of the health care reforms. There has been an ambitious infrastructure building programme and plans to train primary care practitioners. Unfortunately, there has not been a significant increase in visits to primary care as patients still tend to trust hospitals and specialists more. Both the EDL and ZMU policies were first tested at the primary care level. There is evidence of reduced prices and better prescribing, although many facilities have suffered from revenue shortfalls due to decreases in drug revenue. As with hospitals, implementation of ZMU must be accompanied by payment reform that rewards care quality or reforms will be unsustainable and primary care facilities will find ways to "game" more revenue.

Chapter 12: Pharmacies and pharmacists in China. Drug sales have long been dominated by hospitals, but China's pharmacy sector is growing rapidly. The government sees them as another avenue by which the link between drug sales and hospital revenues can be reduced. They can also provide easy access to pharmaceuticals for patients in the community. Retail of pharmaceuticals over the Internet is also growing rapidly, providing an alternative to bricks-and-mortar stores. Pharmacists themselves can play an important role in promoting rational prescribing and in educating patients and providers in both hospitals and the community. Unfortunately, there is a shortage of pharmacists, particularly those who work clinically. More government support is needed to train and regulate pharmacists so that they can play a large role in the health care system.

Chapter 13: Traditional Chinese medicine. Traditional Chinese medicine (TCM), a significant part of health care in China, has been used for thousands of years. TCM incorporates acupuncture and the use of herbal preparations and it is the latter that will be the subject of this discussion. In recent decades, efforts have been made to modernize the field through more rigorous research into active ingredients and mechanisms of action. Most Chinese have used TCM, although western medicine is becoming increasingly popular. This has increased the risk of drug–herb interactions and other adverse drug reactions, particularly as the understanding of many TCMs is quite limited. Regulation of TCM preparations is challenging, as they are innately less standardized and more susceptible to contamination compared with western medications. In spite of these challenges, the popularity of TCM in other countries has helped to drive brisk growth in the export market.

Chapter 14: Industrial policy. China's industrial policy should have the twin objectives of fostering a truly innovative pharmaceutical sector capable of producing novel medications while strengthening a domestic generics industry so that it can provide affordable quality medications. Market fragmentation, driven by local protectionism, is a hallmark of China's pharmaceutical environment and must be addressed to meet either of these objectives. R&D spending has increased rapidly in recent years and many multinational corporations are interested in investing in China. However, overall R&D levels are still much lower than in western countries and an unfavourable policy environment has contributed to low returns on R&D. China must also gradually refine its intellectual property rights regime and continue to fight corruption. China will be most effective in meeting its industrial policy objectives if it is able to incorporate them into a national pharmaceutical strategy that seeks to align reforms in other aspects of pharmaceutical policy, such as drug approvals, pricing and reimbursement.

The final chapter, Chapter 15, outlines the overall conclusions and policy recommendations.

1.3 Report methodology

Four main information streams were used for this report: a systematic–narrative review, a review of Chinese Government documents and statistical handbooks, a series of seminars on pharmaceutical policy, and fieldwork and interviews (Fig. 1.1).

Fig. 1.1 Summary of information sources used in the review

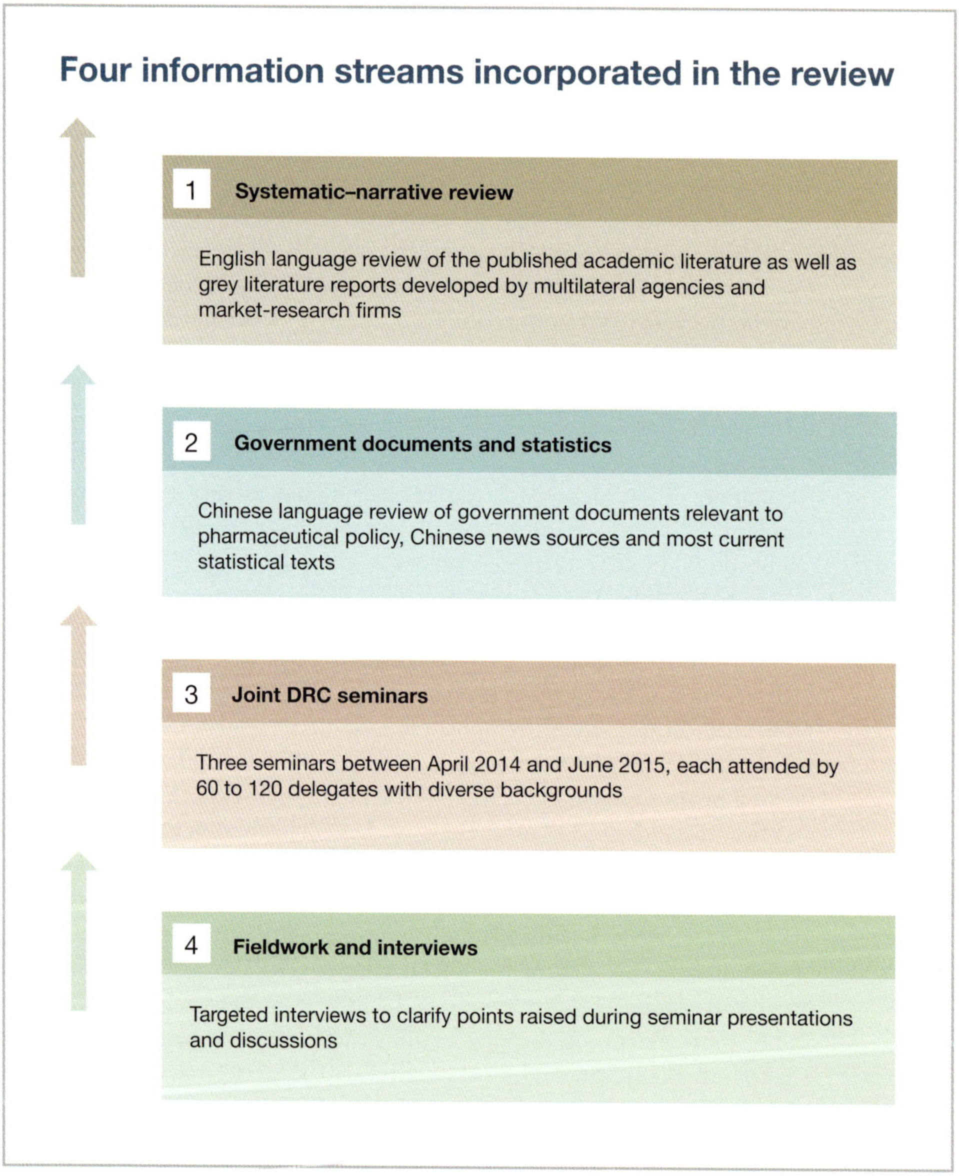

Note: DRC: Development Research Center of the State Council.

A systematic–narrative review was conducted to critically appraise and summarize the evidence on Chinese pharmaceutical policy. Systematic–narrative reviews are a type of systematic literature search that incorporates narrative syntheses and analysis. It was chosen in order to summarize the extensive information available in the academic literature as well as in the grey literature. The review component involved a search of the English academic literature and of the English grey literature. The grey literature search particularly concentrated on reports from market research companies and multilateral agencies. For the academic portion of the review, an English language search for publications published between 2005 and September 2015 was carried out using three databases: MEDLINE (a biomedical database), EconLit (an economics database) and Business Source Premier (a business-oriented database). The specific search terms can be found in Appendix 2. A review of references in key papers was also performed to identify other important publications. The review of grey literature reports was carried out using similar search terms for the period from 2010 to 2015.

The second part of the review involved a Chinese language search of government documents, Chinese news sources and Chinese statistical handbooks. Incorporating these primary sources provided a picture of the current policy milieu and a firm quantitative understanding of China's pharmaceutical environment.

This report also draws on insights and material from presentations in a series of seminars on Chinese pharmaceutical policy organized by the authors' academic department and the Development Research Center of the State Council. There were three seminars: one in April 2014 in Beijing, another in October 2014 in London, and finally one in June 2015 in Beijing. A wide array of Chinese experts representing policy-making bodies, government, universities and industry were in attendance. The list of attendees can be found in Appendix 1.

Following the seminars, the authors engaged in fieldwork by conducting interviews with seminar participants as well as other experts in Chinese pharmaceutical policy. These interviews were used to clarify information from over 40 seminar presentations and their associated discussions. Interviews were conducted in a semistructured fashion, with questions modified depending on the stakeholder being interviewed. For example, agencies involved with health insurance would be asked clarifying questions about coverage levels while those involved with pricing would be asked more about tendering and other pricing policies. A brief interview guide is available upon request. Interviews were conducted in order to clarify and corroborate what was found in written sources. Interviews were also used to identify major gaps in knowledge or to identify key government documents. Information from the seminars and interviews is not attributed to specific individuals as pharmaceutical policy reform is a politically sensitive topic in China.

This report provides an extensive overview of the major issues in Chinese pharmaceutical policy. The information provided is very current and includes the perspectives of important Chinese stakeholders. The report covers both issues that are traditionally related to pharmaceuticals, such as pricing and reimbursement, drug quality, and access and affordability, and also how pharmaceutical policy interacts with the health system at large. This includes the health challenges China will face in the coming decades and how the hospital, primary care and pharmacy systems relate to pharmaceutical policy. There is also a discussion on TCM, which remains an important way by which Chinese acquire health care. Industrial policy – a priority of Chinese leadership – is also discussed. Following the descriptive–analytical presentation of China's pharmaceutical environment in Chapters 2–14, key recommendations for future reforms are also provided in Chapter 15.

2. Introduction to Chinese health care reform and pharmaceutical policy

KEY MESSAGES

- China's health care system is facing significant demographic challenges and a rapidly increasingly prevalence of NCDs.
- Health care reforms during the 1980s and 1990s led to large declines in government funding that were unfortunately replaced with drug sales and increased private spending.
- The 2009 health care reforms, targeted at five priority areas, aim to address problems of cost, equity and efficiency and all have linkages with pharmaceutical policy:
  - expanding insurance coverage rates: remarkable progress has been made but efforts should be made to better harmonize the benefits paid out by the three schemes and to include more migrant workers;
  - strengthening public health services: reorientation of services and health promotion to tackle NCD should be a priority;
  - promoting and strengthening primary care: will improve access, equity and affordability but further government subsidies are needed to train physicians and to make up for lost income from ZMU;
  - public hospital reform: removing the linkage of hospital revenue with drug sales is a difficult but essential component of broader health care reform; and
  - reforming drug policy and implementing the EDL: this has occurred widely and has led to some decreases in drug costs but many problems remain in the overall pharmaceutical environment.
- Effective pharmaceutical reform will require concerted action across all stakeholders, including government, providers, patients and industry. An overarching national pharmaceutical framework could be very helpful in achieving coordinated reform.

2.1 Background to China's health care system

China has experienced historically unprecedented economic growth over the past several decades but this growth has brought with it significant health challenges. China's 1.35 billion people are rapidly ageing, with projections suggesting that by 2050 almost 30% of the population will be over the age of 65 (Mattke et al., 2014). Meanwhile, the prevalence of NCDs such as hypertension and diabetes mellitus is rapidly increasing beyond even levels in developed countries. This demographic and epidemiological shift, coupled with increasing wealth, means there is an enormous demand for health care that is only going to continue to increase. In 2012, China spent 5.4% of its GDP on health (Fig. 2.1), much less than the OECD average of 9.3% (OECD, 2014; WHO, 2014c). Compared with others in the BRICS grouping, China spends proportionally less than Brazil (10%), Russia (7%) and South Africa (9%) but more than India (4%) (OECD, 2014; WHO, 2014c). However, by 2020 China's THE is projected to reach US$ 1 trillion, or 7% of its GDP (Daemmrich, 2013). These figures understate total spending as they exclude some direct patient spending on nursing care as well as any under-the-table payments (Development Research Center of the State Council, 2015). A strong set of pharmaceutical policies is an essential part of a successful health care system and has been, and will continue to be, an integral part of Chinese health policy. The effects of the 2009 reforms on pharmaceutical policy will be explored in this chapter and throughout the report.

2.2 A brief history of health care in China

When the Communist Party took control of China in 1949, it created a successful public health care system. The government owned, funded and staffed all health care institutions from small rural clinics to large urban hospitals, and all physicians were employees of the state. At the time, most Chinese lived in the countryside and so health care was organized by the same communes that owned the land and organized farming (Blumenthal & Hsiao, 2005). The much-vaunted barefoot doctors, health cadres who received basic training, staffed these commune-run health centres. There was also a strong public health apparatus that engaged in activities such as widespread immunization campaigns and the promotion of better sanitation. From 1950 to 1982, huge strides were made in life expectancy, increasing from 42.2 to 64.4 years. During this time, infant mortality also fell by 75%, from the 130s to the 30s per 1000 births (Brown et al., 2012)

In the early 1980s, in conjunction with Deng Xiaoping's market liberalization reforms, the government relinquished many of its health care responsibilities almost overnight. From 1978 to 1999, the central government's share of THE fell from 32% to 15% (National Health Development Research Center, 2013). The burden of spending fell upon provinces and individuals, with OOP expenditure as a share of total health care spending increasing from 20% in 1978 to 58% in 2001 (National Health Development Research Center, 2013). As the government withdrew funding, barefoot doctors became unemployed and money for public health activities plummeted. This led to a collapse of China's formerly strong primary care and public health system. The rural health care insurance programme that had previously existed also collapsed and by 1999 only 7% of

Fig. 2.1 Health expenditure as share of GDP in China and OECD countries

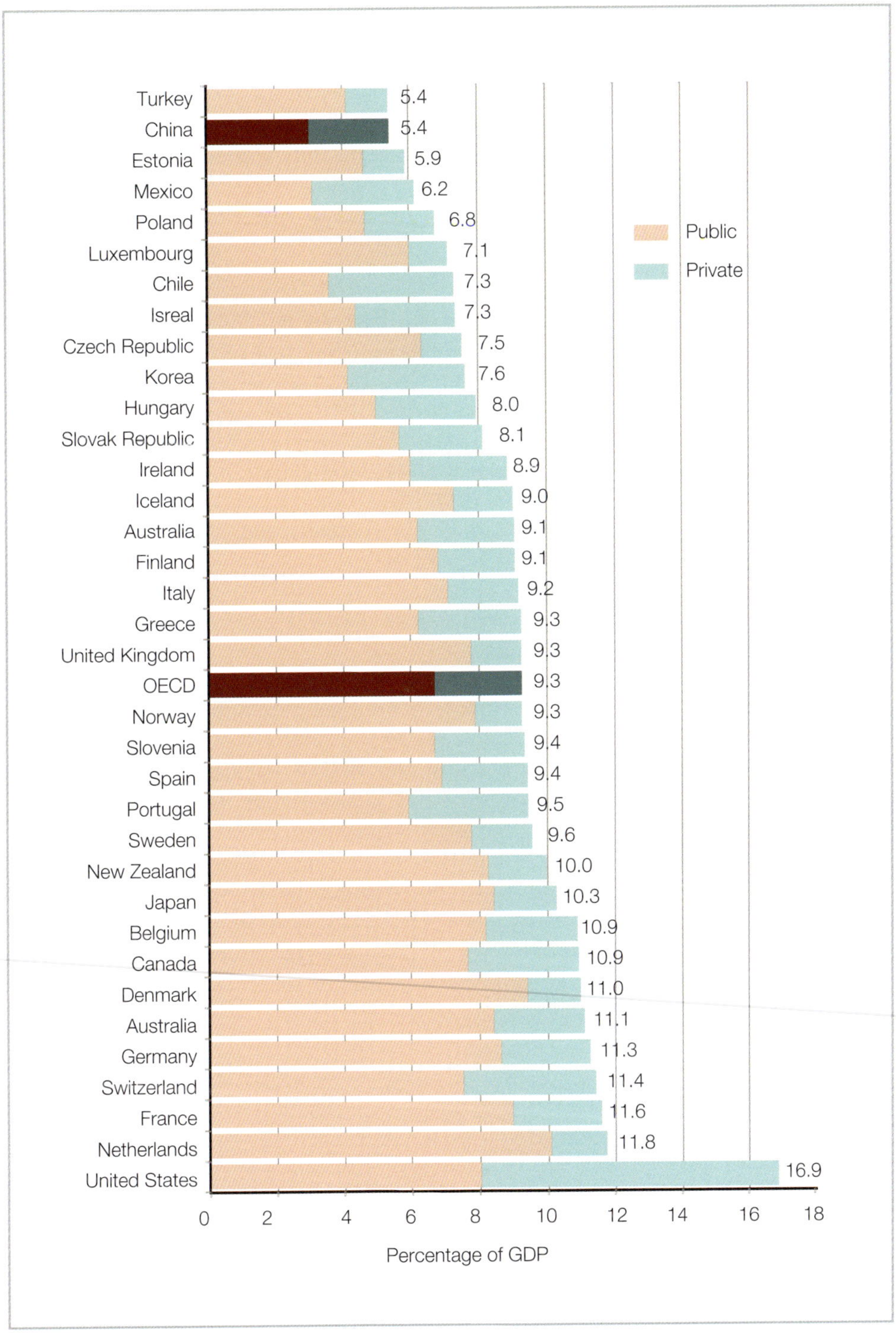

Sources: OECD, 2014; WHO, 2014c.

rural residents had any form of insurance. In larger hospitals, the government stipulated that funding shortfalls could be covered by charging a 15% mark-up on sales of medications, devices and diagnostic testing, and doctors and hospitals could earn revenue from this mark-up. The 15% mark-up policy incentivized expensive, often irrational, treatment and led to significantly negative consequences for pharmaceutical policy. China's spending on pharmaceuticals as a percentage of THE was 37.6% in 2011 (Center for Health Statistics and Information, 2013), much higher than the OECD average of 19% (OECD, 2013a).

2.3 Health care reforms launched

Following widespread discontent at the state of health care in China, the central government unveiled significant reforms in April 2009 with the goal of "providing affordable and equitable basic health care for all by 2020". The reforms were centred on five priority areas:

- expand insurance coverage with a target of establishing universal coverage by 2011;
- strengthen public health services through government spending, especially in lower-income areas;
- promote and establish primary care facilities that will serve as gatekeepers to the health care system in the long-run;
- encourage public hospital reform through promotion of pilot projects; and
- reform the pharmaceutical market and develop a list of national essential medicines.

The government committed an initial RMB 850 billion investment for the health care reforms. Generally, health care spending growth has exceeded overall GDP growth in the past few years but there is significant variation, ranging from a year-on-year growth rate of 21.4% in 2009 to only 6.8% in 2010 (Fig. 2.2) (National Health Development Research Center, 2013). In terms of the reform goals, the government has achieved some successes but has much to do in order to reach its goal of affordable and equitable basic health care for all.

Expanding insurance coverage

The government has been quite successful at expanding coverage rates. In 2003, only 21% of rural residents had insurance but by 2011 97.5% of rural residents (and 95% of the total population) had access to health insurance (Chen, 2012). Coverage is provided through three major insurance schemes: the Urban Employee Basic Medical Insurance (UEBMI) for formal sector urban workers and retirees, the URBMI for other urban residents and the NCMS for rural residents. While coverage rates are quite high, the quantity of coverage varies dramatically. Both reimbursement rates and reimbursement ceilings are much higher in the UEBMI than in the NCMS (Table 2.1) (Barber & Yao, 2010; Hsiao,

Fig. 2.2 Percentage growth in health care expenditures and overall GDP, 2000–2012

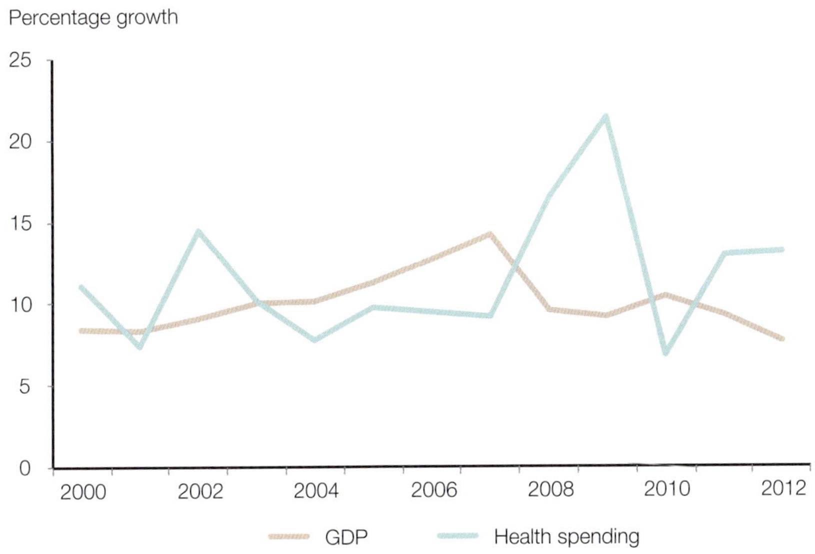

Source: National Health Development Research Center, 2013.

Li & Zhang, 2014; Meng et al., 2015; Niu, 2015; Yip et al., 2012). For example, co-payments for inpatient care for the NCMS can be up to 25–35% and OOP payments can be as high as 90% for some conditions (McKinsey, 2012). The new 2015 State Council work plan calls for higher minimum reimbursement rates (70–80% of inpatient expenses) (State Council, 2015d). Differential coverage levels have significant implications for what drugs are reimbursed and the extent to which they are reimbursed across the country.

While there has been a significant decline in the percentage of OOP expenditures, from 56% to 36%, between 2003 and 2011 (Center for Health Statistics and Information, 2013), surveys have shown that about half of Chinese people feel that affordability has not improved (Deloitte, 2011). Insurance is also not easily portable, and many of China's over 260 million migrant workers do not receive health care benefits (The Wall Street Journal, 2015). This is because their health insurance is linked to their place of official residence, the rural areas that they come from, and they are not eligible for UEBMI coverage in the cities they work in. In summary, China has been successful at creating a highly inclusive insurance scheme but will need to increase benefits, particularly in rural areas and for migrant workers, if it is to properly address the issue of rising medical costs.

Table 2.1 Comparison of China's three main insurance schemes

Insurance scheme	Annual contributions	Approximate coverage levels for medical services and drugs	Annual coverage ceilings
NCMS	Individual: US$ 18.7 (RMB 120) Central government: US$ 59.3 (RMB 380) Regional government: highly variable depending on local income	Inpatient: 55% Outpatient: 50%	Eight times income of local farmers
URBMI	Individual: varies by region Central government: US$ 43.7 (RMB 280) Regional government: highly variable depending on local income	Inpatient: 55% Outpatient: 50%	Six times disposable income of local residents
UEBMI	8% of employee wages: 6% from payroll tax on employers and 2% employee contribution Part of the contribution goes to medical savings account for outpatient expenses and part goes to a larger insurance pool for inpatient expenses	Inpatient: 75% Outpatient: use of medical savings account (limited pooling of funds)	Six times average wage of employee in city

Sources: Barber & Yao, 2010; Hsiao, Li & Zhang, 2014; Meng et al., 2015; Niu, 2015; Yip et al., 2012.

Strengthening public health services

China has enjoyed notable public health successes, such as a widespread vaccination campaign against hepatitis B that significantly decreased prevalence of this once very common disease (Chee, Xie & Nakhimovsky, 2012). However, the burden of diseases is rapidly transitioning to NCDs such as diabetes, cardiovascular diseases and cancer. The focus of China's public health activities must pivot to improving management of NCDs. For example, a recent study highlighted that without better smoking cessation efforts, 3 million Chinese will die every year from smoking by 2050 (Chen et al., 2015).

In 2011, the government announced funding of RMB 25 per person dedicated to public health activities, including health records, health promotion, vaccination, maternal child health, mental health and NCDs. This has gradually been increased to RMB 40 per person as of 2015 (qqjjsj.com, 2015). However, far more needs to be done to help to strengthen China's public health infrastructure from both an investment and a policy perspective. Pharmaceutical policies that make medications for the management of chronic conditions affordable and accessible will be an important part of dealing with the major public health threat posed by NCDs. China has a long way to go if it is to have an effective public health system that is capable of addressing the upstream causes of NCDs through health promotion and protection activities.

Promoting primary care

A strong primary care system is important in creating equitable access and cutting costs, particularly in China's current specialist-driven system where patients will go to tertiary hospitals for minor issues. Lack of trust in the primary care system may be one of the most difficult challenges to overcome in primary care reform. China is looking to reduce the number of outpatient visits at specialized city hospitals and to increase the two-way referral pathways between hospitals and primary care clinics (State Council, 2015a).

The government has committed to building urban community health centres (CHCs) and rural township health centres (THCs) and training primary care staff. They hope to train 300 000 general practitioners within the next 10 years with a target of 2 or 3 for every 10 000 residents (Liu et al., 2011). Given that all of England has only slightly more than 40 000 general practitioners (Anderson, 2013), these are hugely ambitious goals. China's EDL, discussed below, was introduced at the primary care level. The EDL was introduced in tandem with the ZMU policy and aimed to eliminate the 15% mark-ups that health care facilities are able to charge.

Public hospital reform

China is overly reliant on hospitals for providing all forms of health care provision. They are the most common place for patients to access care. China's over 20 000 hospitals (Table 2.2) account for a large percentage of inpatient and outpatient visits in spite of efforts to strengthen the primary care system (Center for Health Statistics and Information, 2013). Overutilization of hospitals and underutilization of primary care is a very inefficient mechanism for health care delivery.

Many of the problems with China's health care system are manifest in hospitals, for example overprescribing of drugs as a result of misaligned incentives, lack of sufficient coverage for catastrophic illness and overreliance on specialists for even simple conditions. Building an effective and rational health care system necessitates effective public hospital reform, given their huge role in the provision of patient care.

Among urban hospitals, a first wave of pilot projects was launched in 16 cities covering a range of reforms from removing the link between drug sales and revenues to increasing

Table 2.2 Number and type of hospitals in China

Insurance	2005	2008	2009	2010	2011	2012
By economic classification[a]						
Public	15483	14309	14051	13850	13539	13384
Non-public	3220	5403	6240	7068	8440	9786
By hospital level[b]						
Tier 3	946	1192	1233	1284	1399	1624
Tier 2	5156	6780	6523	6472	6468	6566
Tier 1	2714	4989	5110	5271	5636	5962
Total	18703	19712	20291	20918	21979	23170

Source: Center for Health Statistics and Information, 2013.

Notes: [a] Public hospitals tend to be much larger than non-public;
[b] China ranks its hospitals by tiers, with Tier 3 being the largest and most complex.

private ownership to the introduction of standardized clinical pathways. A second wave of pilot reforms was announced in 2014 for another 17 cities. Meanwhile, reforms have been gradually increasing among county hospitals, with about half of China's county hospitals having introduced ZMU (Ellis, 2015; State Council, 2015d).

Crucial aspects of hospital reform related to pharmaceutical policy include broader implementation of the ZMU policy and commensurate increases in funding to make up for revenue lost from drug sales and the expansion of the EDL to higher-tier hospitals (the tier system indicating increasing functional levels, tier 3 being the most advanced).

Drug reform and the national EDL

The importance of pharmaceutical policy to health care is reflected in the fact that it is one of the five reform pillars. There are many issues with the current environment, including the 15% mark-up policy, which drives expensive and irrational prescribing; problems in safety and quality from a fragmented manufacturing and supply chain; constantly evolving and variable pricing and reimbursement mechanisms; and incoherent industrial policy. The reforms also specifically called for the creation of an EDL.

The lack of a national pharmaceutical policy framework is a major barrier to coherent and coordinated reforms. There is significant regulatory fragmentation in China and forums for communication across partners are quite weak. This has led to significant policy variation across different Chinese provinces. Finally, there is limited monitoring of new and existing pharmaceutical policies. This is particularly problematic given the rate at which new policies are being announced.

While this report focuses on western prescription medications, TCM and over-the-counter (OTC) medicines are also important parts of China's pharmaceutical market. TCM has been used in China for thousands of years. Recently, the Chinese Government has pursued a modernization agenda to improve the quality and standardization of TCM as well as our scientific understanding for its use. TCM accounts for about 30% of total pharmaceutical spending and about half of OTC spending. More than a third of China's EDL and larger NRDL is made up of TCM preparations. There are significant challenges in guaranteeing the safety of TCMs because of their heterogeneous nature, the potential for contamination and interactions between TCMs and other medications.

OTC medicines, including both western and TCM drugs, make up 18% of total pharmaceutical sales in China (China Nonprescription Medicines Association, 2012). Unlike prescription drugs, OTC medications are sold primarily in retail pharmacies rather than hospitals, in approximately a three to two ratio (China Nonprescription Medicines Association, 2012). The EDL contains 175 (34%) OTC medications of which 60 are western drugs and 175 are TCM preparations. Sales growth in OTC medications have been in the double digits but have been lower than for prescription drugs. The most popular OTC drugs are for colds/coughs/allergies, lifestyle regulation (includes sedatives, contraceptives, smoking cessation, diet drugs, etc.) and vitamins/minerals/supplements (China Nonprescription Medicines Association, 2012). As with prescription drugs, OTC drugs are regulated by the CFDA. OTC drugs are divided into class A drugs, which require a pharmaceutical enterprise permit to be sold, and class B drugs, which do not have this requirement. As with any medication, OTC drugs can interact with other medications and lead to adverse health outcomes. Consequently, improving the ability of pharmacists and physicians to identify such interactions is important in ensuring patient safety.

2.4 Conclusions

China has made significant strides in improving its health care system following the 2009 reforms: insurance coverage rates are close to 100%; the EDL has been established and is being used across the country; and primary care is gradually being strengthened. As to be expected, huge challenges remain in reforming a health care system that serves so many people in such a short period of time. Effective pharmaceutical policies will be essential in ensuring that the broader health care reforms are successful in achieving equitable and affordable basic health care.

3. Regulatory structure and drug approval

KEY MESSAGES

- Responsibility for health care in China is spread across many different ministries, commissions and organizations at the national level. Provincial and local agencies can also exert considerable influence. This leads to problems with fragmentation and a lack of transparency.
- There is no national pharmaceutical strategy that coordinates the actions of all the government organizations involved in the pharmaceutical market.
- Key players include the National Health and Family Planning Commission (NHFPC; overall guidance of reforms, manages EDL and NCMS), the National Development and Reform Commission (NDRC; pricing), the Ministry of Human Resources and Social Security (manages URBMI, UEBMI and NRDL) and the CFDA.
- The CFDA is responsible for new drug approvals and the monitoring of drug quality. There have been many reforms introduced recently aimed at improving the drug approvals and market authorization process.
- There is a significant backlog of almost 19 000 applications at the CFDA. This is partly driven by the large number of "me-too" generic applicants coming from China's fragmented pharmaceutical manufacturing industry but also by a lack of effective signalling mechanisms to guide which drugs should receive priority approval.
- Increasing the human resources and institutional capacity of the CFDA and its provincial affiliates is essential in ensuring that NDAs are reviewed in a timely fashion and the quality of drugs can be effectively monitored.

3.1 Health care governance and regulation

Responsibility for health care is fragmented across various government ministries, all of which fall under the supervision of China's State Council, the country's highest executive body. The key ministries involved in health care are the NHFPC, the NDRC and the Ministry of Human Resources and Social Security. Other ministries involved in health care include the Ministries of Finance, Civil Affairs, Industry and Information Technology, and Commerce and the Chinese Insurance Regulatory Commission (Fig. 3.1) (NDRC, 2014b; State Council, 2015f; Yip et al., 2012).

Fig. 3.1 Key ministries and organizations involved in Chinese health care

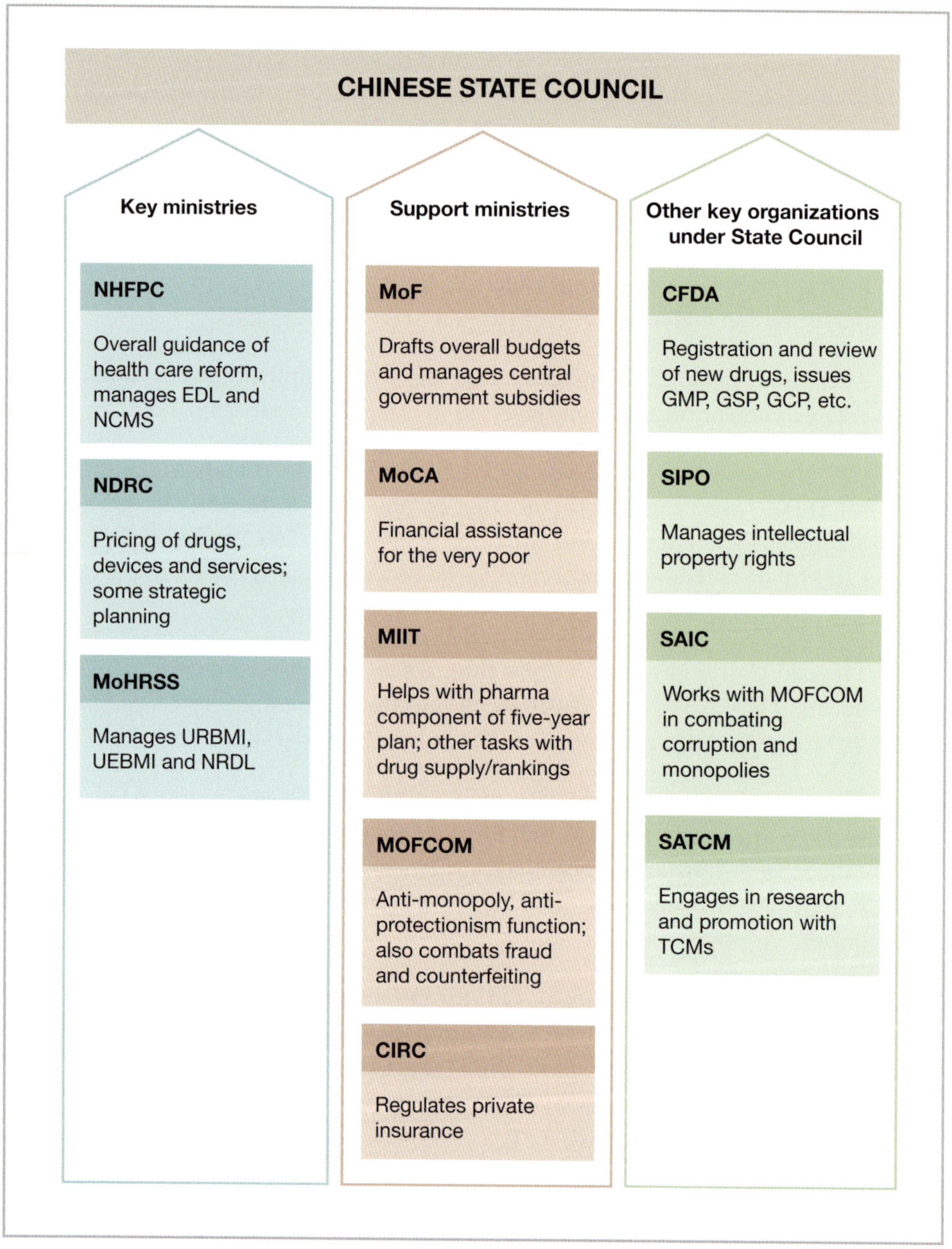

Sources: NDRC, 2014b; State Council, 2015f; Yip et al., 2012.

Notes: CIRC: Chinese Insurance Regulatory Commission; GCP: Good Clinical Practice; GSP: Good Supply Practice; MIIT: Ministry of Industry and Information Technology; MoCA: Ministry of Civil Affairs; MoF: Ministry of Finance; MOFCOM: Ministry of Commerce; MoHRSS: Ministry of Human Resources and Social Security; SAIC: State Administration for Industry and Commerce; SATM: State Administration of Traditional Chinese Medicine; SIPO: State Intellectual Property Office.

Key ministries

NHFPC. Formed through the merger of the Ministry of Health and the National Family Planning Commission in 2013, this is the agency most responsible for health care. Responsibilities include overall guidance for health care reform; management of the EDL, including drug selection and tendering; administration of the NCMS; and promotion of public hospital and primary care reform.

NDRC. The key responsibility of the NDRC is in monitoring, forecasting and regulating prices of drugs, medical devices and medical services. It contains the High-technology Industry Office, which plans strategic development of new industries. Up to June 2015, it also used to set price ceilings for medications, which were abolished.

Ministry of Human Resources and Social Security. This ministry manages the URBMI and UEBMI schemes and is also responsible for the NRDL.

Supporting ministries

Ministry of Finance. The Ministry of Finance drafts budgets for the NHFPC, the Ministry of Human Resources and Social Security and the Ministry of Civil Affairs. It also manages the central government's subsidies to local government to support health care and collects information on various health insurance schemes.

Ministry of Civil Affairs. The Ministry has responsible for maintaining a social safety net for the most poor in urban and rural areas, a role which extends into access to health care.

Ministry of Industry and Information Technology. The pharmaceutical component of the 12th Five Year Plan is implemented by this Ministry, which also compiles rankings of pharmaceutical companies to be used for tendering. The Ministry issues the vaccine production plan, strengthens management of basic drug supply and oversees structural adjustment of the pharmaceutical industry.

Ministry of Commerce. The main role of the Ministry of Commerce in health care is through the Antimonopoly Bureau and the Market Order Office, both of which are responsible for challenging monopolies, dealing with regional protectionism and working with other departments to fight intellectual property rights infringement, counterfeiting and other types of fraud. The Ministry also regulates imports and exports, which has bearing on imported drugs.

Chinese Insurance Regulatory Commission. The Commission is responsible for the regulation of commercial health insurance.

Other key government agencies

CFDA. As the primary pharmaceutical regulator, the CFDA plays an essential role. It is responsible for the registration and review of drugs, medical devices, foods and cosmetics in China. It contains the Center for Drug Evaluation (CDE), which is the technical review arm of the CFDA. It issues policies on GMP and Good Laboratory Practice and also regulations for Good Supply Practice and Good Clinical Practice. It conducts inspections to ensure compliance. It sets practice standards for clinical pharmacists, is responsible for their registration and is also responsible for regulation of TCM.

State Intellectual Property Office. The Office manages patents and intellectual property in China and implements court decisions in patent and intellectual property disputes.

State Administration for Industry and Commerce. This assists the Ministry of Commerce in fighting monopolies, unfair competitive practices and illegal practices, including bribery and smuggling.

State Administration of Traditional Chinese Medicine. This is the agency responsible for coordinating and promoting the R&D of TCM and in formulating TCM-related policies.

Non-State Council actors

It is important to mention the role of two non-State Council actors. The Supreme People's Procuratorate is China's highest judicial body and contains within it the Anti-Corruption Office, which deals with bribery and graft, embezzlement of public funds and other acts of corruption and criminal activity. The People's Liberation Army, China's armed forces, runs a number of military hospitals throughout the country. In addition to these central actors, there are various provincial counterparts that can exert considerable influence. For example, there are provincial health and family planning commissions, development and reform commissions, food and drug administrations and ministries of human resources and social services.

3.2 Challenges to health care governance

Different ministries responsible for health care often have conflicting priorities. Horizontal fragmentation at the level of central government and vertical fragmentation between the central and provincial governments create coordination barriers to policy formulation and implementation. For example, at the central level the Ministry of Finance is required to approve large funding requests and it can be reluctant to provide what is requested by health officials. In addition, while overall guidance for tendering and procurement is provided at a national level, provinces have significant discretion with implementation, leading to dramatic differences in actual policy implementation.

Significant regulatory fragmentation also contributes to a lack of transparency in policy-making. This translates into a perceived lack of consultation and forward guidance for domestic and foreign drug manufacturers (Development Research Center of the State Council, 2015). All these factors mean that the policy envisioned by government officials is often very different from the policy that is implemented on the ground. Uncertainty can be found in all areas of pharmaceutical policy, including drug approvals, quality standards, and pricing and reimbursement, creating a climate that can be difficult for manufacturers to negotiate. Furthermore, limited data are available on overall prescribing practices and spending that could be used to improve guidance and effectively evaluate reforms.

Corruption is another major problem in China, occurring at both government and hospital/physician levels. In 2007, the head of the State Food and Drug Administration, the predecessor to the CFDA, was executed for taking bribes in the drug approval process (Yu et al., 2010). In 2013, GlaxoSmithKline received record fines for bribing government officials and physicians to promote sales of their drugs (Jia, 2013). In response to the widespread outrage at corruption in health care that emerged from this event, the NHFPC issued "Prohibition on 9 unethical conducts to strengthen morals in the health-care industry", which banned physicians from taking kickbacks from patients or companies (NHFPC, 2013a). Although reform efforts are ongoing, the culture of bribing and paying kickbacks to physicians to sell drugs or devices has been entrenched in China for a long time and will be difficult to remove. There is also a culture of cronyism in which state-owned pharmaceutical firms are often run by former government officials. These officials are able to extend significant protection to these firms. This protectionism is a well-recognized problem that contributes to problems in improving China's pharmaceutical industrial policy.

3.3 Drug approval pathways in China

Legislation for the current drug approval pathways in China is set out in the Drug Registration Regulation, which debuted in 2007 and was amended in 2013 (McTiernan, 2015c). In general, the process for new drug approval is based on the pathway used by the US FDA (PPD, 2013). Clinical trials require a clinical trial application, which is similar to the United States investigational new drug system. After trials are complete, companies are then able to submit an NDA for review. NDAs are reviewed by the CDE, the CFDA's technical arm. The CFDA has its own standards for Good Clinical Practice, Good Laboratory Practice and GMP. While these standards have gradually been improving since their establishment in 1999, they do not yet reach international standards (PPD, 2013).

There are various pathways for NDAs in China. Broadly speaking, applications are classified into chemical drugs, biologicals and TCMs. Domestically produced drugs (innovative or generic) first seek approval through a provincial food and drug administration unit and then require CFDA approval, while drugs from international companies go directly through the CFDA (Yan, 2013). The vast majority of applications to the CFDA are for chemical drugs, which will be the focus of this chapter. Very recently, the CFDA did release guidelines for the evaluation of biosimilars, a market with huge potential in China (McTiernan, 2015b). For chemical drugs, there are six different application pathways (categories; Table 3.1) (PPD, 2013).

Table 3.1 Drug approval pathways for chemical drugs in China

Category	Description
I	New drug not yet approved in any other jurisdiction
II	Drug seeking approval for a new route of administration not approved in any other jurisdiction
III	Drug approved in other countries but not in China
IV	Drug made by changing the acidic or alkaline radicals or metallic elements of the salt of a drug approved in China without changing original pharmacological effects
V	Changed dosage form of a drug approved in China without changing the route of administration
VI	Generic drug with existing national standards in China

Source: PPD, 2013.

The most commonly sought out pathways are I, III, VI and a hybrid of I and III – multiregional clinical trials (Fig. 3.2). Note with the global application scenario, companies develop a new medication completely outside of China, obtain a certificate of pharmaceutical product and then are able to seek approval within China via a category III application (Su, 2013).

Category I applications involve carrying out the entire drug development process in China and are the most resource intensive. Category III applications require fewer resources but can only be initiated when the global certificate of pharmaceutical product has been obtained. Multiregional clinical trial applications are a hybrid of I and III and are increasingly popular, but recently the government has required an additional clinical trial application after a certificate of pharmaceutical product is given and before the NDA, causing significant delays (McTiernan, 2014c). Lastly, category VI applications require a form of limited bioequivalence testing (and even this was not required prior to 2007). Companies face significant delays in waiting for the CFDA to approve both new and generic medications because of the large number of applications every year, a significant existing backlog and insufficient staff to deal with the workload.

In November of 2015, the CFDA proposed a new draft document calling for the creation of new registration categories for chemical drugs (CFDA, 2015a). Under the proposed system, there will be five categories for new drug registrations. Categories I and II will be for innovative drugs not marketed anywhere and for "improved" drugs not marketed

Fig. 3.2 Requirements for most common drug approval pathways in China

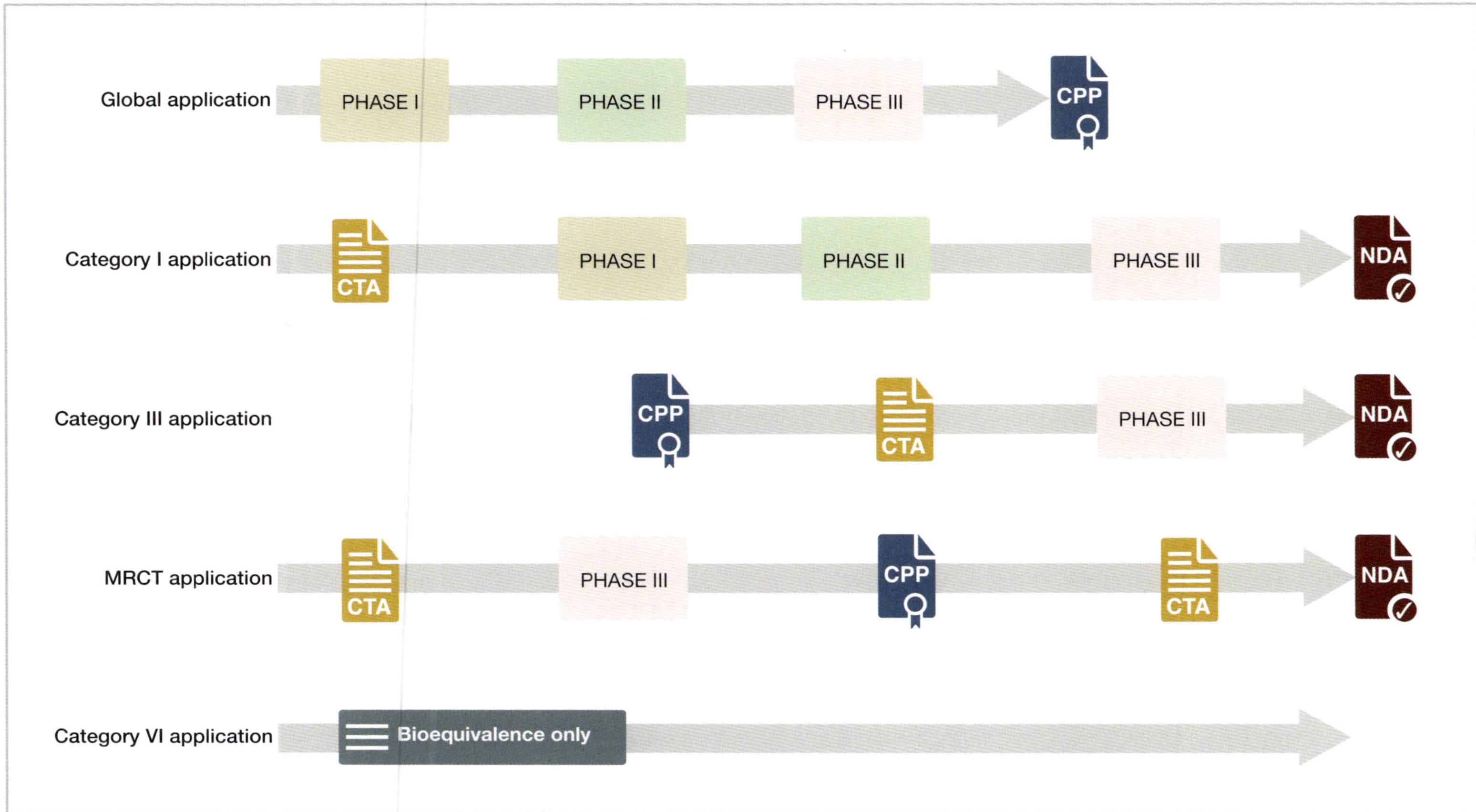

Notes: CPP: Certificate of pharmaceutical product; CTA: Clinical trial application; MRCT: Multiregional clinical trial.

anywhere (i.e. changes in structure, dosage form, route of administration and so on that have clear clinical benefit), respectively. Categories III through V would be for generic medicines – essentially defined drugs that are already sold elsewhere. Interestingly, this means that on-patent drugs marketed abroad but not in China would enter as a category 3 generic rather than a category I or II innovative drug.

The National People's Congress also announced a pilot scheme for a market authorization holder system for drug manufacturers that would be more in line with that used in developed countries (National People's Congress, 2015). Under China's current system, receiving market authorization is contingent on having a manufacturing facility capable of actually producing the drug. This has limited the ability of R&D organizations such as universities from commercializing the drugs they develop and has led to an excessive amount of manufacturing capacity.

3.4 Drug approval delays

Delays in drug approvals are becoming increasingly problematic in China. According to the 2014 CDE annual report, there were 8868 registration applications, of which 7829 were for chemical drugs (CDE, 2015). This brought the total backlog of applications to 18 597 by the end of 2014, an increase of over 4000 from the previous year (Fig. 3.3) (CDE, 2015). This means that novel drugs that are clinically superior to existing treatments or generic medications for drugs that are coming off-patent are not approved in a

Fig. 3.3 New applications, completed applications and backlog for review, 2011–2014

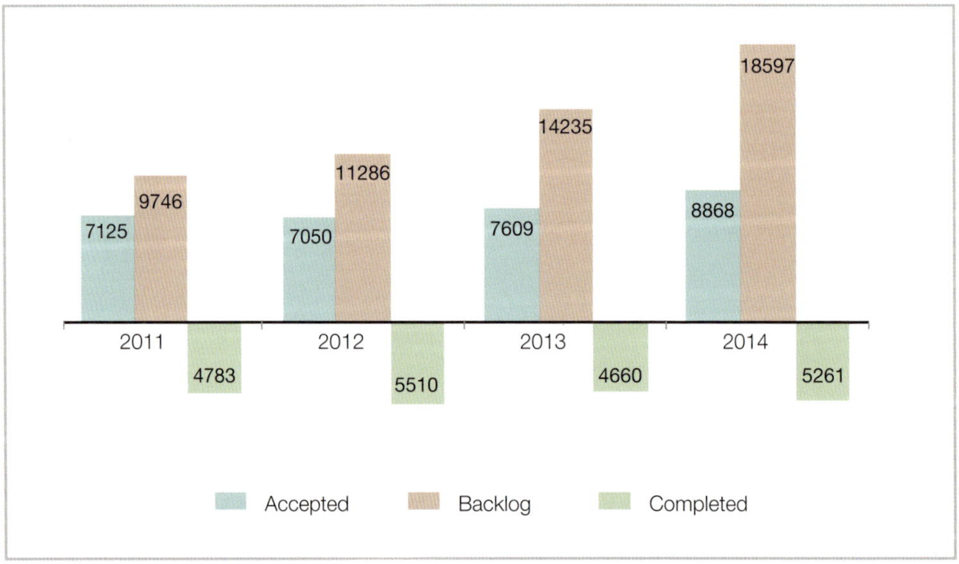

Source: CDE, 2015.

timely fashion. As a result, China loses out on the clinical benefits of new drugs and the cost savings of actually needed generics that do not have dozens of imitators already on market.

Part of the reason there are such significant delays is the very limited human resource capacity of the CDE. The organization has only 89 employees to review and approve all NDAs in China. In comparison, the US FDA has over 3000 employees working in this area, which highlights the disparity between the two organizations (US FDA, 2013).

Another reason for the large backlog comes from the submission of identical generics. The CDE report shows that for eight compounds (including the very commonly prescribed esomeprazole, atorvastatin and clopidogrel) there are more than 100 different applications. For many other compounds, there are 10 or more identical generics seeking approval (Table 3.2) (CDE, 2015). Hundreds of submissions for identical molecules is a product of China's highly fragmented drug manufacturing industry, where there are thousands of companies who face limited barriers in submitting applications for generic drugs. Another factor contributing to the approvals lag is the lack of HTA or CER during the approvals process. Both could help to signal which drugs should receive priority review, thereby lessening the time it would take novel compounds or generics for drug just coming off-patent to come on market.

Table 3.2 Number of applications for a given generic molecule

No. applications	No. molecules
>100	8
50–99	23
30–49	30
20–29	51
10–19	115
<10	834

Source: CDE, 2015.

The backlog of work has led to an estimated review time of 10–18 months for a clinical trial application and 12 to 15 months for an NDA (Su, 2013). This is significantly longer than the average review times of other countries. Even after a new drug has been approved, it can still take upwards of four to five years to gain placement on a reimbursement list, further delaying clinical uptake.

Attempts have been made to address this lag and the need to expedite approval of new breakthrough drugs and essential generics. In 2009, the predecessor to the CFDA announced a "Special Review and Approval" regulation that allowed for the fast tracking of new chemical entities, drugs that had previously not been approved in China, and drugs for serious conditions such as human immunodeficiency virus (HIV) infection and the acquired immunodeficiency syndrome (AIDS) and cancer (Su, 2013). A draft amendment to the Drug Registration Regulations in 2013 sought to streamline the drug approval process through the introduction of a Bolar-like provision to encourage the development of new generics (Covington, 2013).

In 2015 the CDE announced significant increases in NDA fees of up to five times. This should help to deter spurious applications from generic manufacturers while increasing the CDE's capacity to review drugs through hiring more staff (McTiernan, 2015c). In the United States, the Prescription Drug User Fee Act, introduced in 1992, helped to address some of the delays in drug approvals they were confronting by charging higher fees from drug companies and channelling it into increased capacity for the US FDA.

In August 2015 the State Council launched a significant overhaul of the drug approval and quality process with a goal of clearing the drug approval backlog by the end of 2016 and of having approvals follow specified timelines by 2018 (CFDA, 2015b; State Council, 2015c). The CFDA also called for stricter criteria for the review and approval of "new" drugs with only minor changes in an effort to stop companies from seeking patent protection for drugs with minimal clinical benefit. As part of the stricter approval standards, the CFDA recently rejected applications for 11 medicines because of inadequacies with clinical trial data (Hirschler & Jourdan, 2015).

At the same time, the CFDA also promised to create a system for the rapid evaluation of innovative drugs for HIV/AIDS, cancer, major chronic diseases, orphan diseases and drugs of significant economic interest to China. Promises have also been made about greater transparency in the approvals process, including clear documentation of requirements and timelines. Unfortunately, targets for approval time remain nebulous or weak, with the CFDA stating that clinical trial applications must be approved only within three years prior to patent expiration. All-in-all, there has been a flurry of policy announcements during 2014 and 2015 that touch on market approval, drug quality and drug pricing (Box 3.1). Hopefully the government's renewed commitment to rationalizing pharmaceutical policy will yield results.

Box 3.1 New pharmaceutical policies in China

During 2014 and 2015, Chinese pharmaceutical policy has evolved at a breakneck pace. There have been a number of hugely significant announcements, some of which are described below.

Drug pricing and tendering

Starting from May 2014, these policies have sought to reform the way in which drugs are priced by abolishing price ceilings, reaffirming tendering as the primary vehicle for pricing and rationalizing and improving the tendering process.

Notice of the NDRC on the abolishment of drug price documents, No. 918. Released in 2014, this policy called for the repeal of the drug price ceilings that have been in place for decades. This policy set the stage for further reform of China's drug pricing and reimbursement system.

Notice of the NDRC on enhancing supervision of drug market pricing activities, No. 830. This was released in conjunction with the above document and called for careful monitoring of drug prices following the lifting of price ceilings to monitor for excessive price jumps or anticompetitive behaviour.

State Council notice of the promulgation of the opinions on advancing drug price reform, No. 7 and State Council notice on implementing and improving centralized bidding and procurement of drugs, No. 7. These two documents, issued in February 2015, outlined the new pricing mechanisms following abolishment of price ceilings. Highlights included the use of tendering as the primary pricing mechanism for off-patent drugs, the use of price negotiations for patented drugs and the introduction of reimbursement caps (a form of IRP). The second of these two documents focused specifically on tendering and touched on issues of tendering by quality group, secondary negotiation and how to create a more unified, transparent system.

NHFPC notice on implementing and improving centralized bidding and procurement of drugs, No. 70. This document was issued a few months following the State Council No. 7 documents (NHFPC, 2015). It called for hospitals to acquire 80% of their medications through the tendering process, for drug sales to not exceed 25–30% of total hospital revenue and for the creation of a more interconnected, transparent tender system

Drug approvals and quality

During 2015, China made several announcements aimed at increasing drug quality, clearing the drug backlog at the CFDA and expediting the approval of important medications.

Announcement of CFDA on soliciting public opinions regarding policies to expedite the reduction of drug registration application backlog, No. 140. Released in July 2015, this document called for bioequivalence testing of generic drugs against a reference drug (which is not done in China), limiting the approval of drugs that have only minor changes made to them and severe consequences for submitting fraudulent application data.

Opinions of the State Council on reforming the evaluation and approval system for drugs and medical devices, No. 44. Released a week after CFDA No. 140, this reiterated many of its points and called for loss of registration for generics that did not meet bioequivalence testing, strict limits to the number of identical generic drugs seeking approval and reaffirmation of fast-track approval pathways for important and novel drugs (State Council, 2015c).

Other policies. Other key policies in the drug approvals domain that have been released recently have been the introduction of a pilot scheme of a market authorization holder system, a proposed change in the categories drugs can apply for and a significant increase in the fees charged by NDAs. There have been many more policies that focus on other aspects of the health care system such as hospital reform and also have significant pharmaceutical ramifications, including broader roll-out of the ZMU policy and limits on the proportion of total revenues hospitals can derive from drug sales.

3.5 Conclusions

China's health care regulatory framework is fragmented and complex. There are many ministries, commissions and other organizations that are involved in health care, each with its own responsibilities. In addition to the large number of organizations present at the national level, there are also provincial and local agencies that are involved. This organizational patchwork contributes to regulatory fragmentation and a lack of transparency that makes coordinated policy-making challenging. Corruption in governments and hospitals is another endemic problem that China's health care reformers must address.

When it comes to China's drug approval process, the CFDA and the CDE are burdened with a huge workload. Excessive market fragmentation leading to too many companies filing NDAs, minimal barriers in applying for new drugs and a lack of evidence-based HTA or CER to guide the approvals process have all led to a significant backlog of NDAs. The backlog delays the approval of novel therapies that could improve health and of generics for newly off-patent drugs that could save the health care system money. The government has been cognizant of these problems and announced in 2015 a series of sweeping regulatory reforms including re-categorizing how drugs are approved, a pilot market authorisation holder system, increased capacity for the CFDA through higher user fees and an overarching promise to expedite the drug approval process. Hopefully, moving forwards China can develop a more coherent national approach to pharmaceutical policy and continue introducing policies that rationalize the drug approval process.

4. Key health issues: ageing, urbanization and noncommunicable diseases

KEY MESSAGES

- Health conditions in China have been improving rapidly over the past several decades. However, China's health system must confront new challenges with changing demographics and an epidemiological transition towards chronic diseases.
- In particular, ageing, urbanization and higher rates of NCDs such as diabetes, cardiovascular diseases and cancer are increasing China's health burden:
  - by 2050, over 30% of China's population will be over the age of 60, higher than the projected OECD average;
  - China has experienced the world's largest urban migration and rapid growth of cities is putting pressure on the health care system;
  - one third of the world's smokers are in China and smoking rates are far higher than in most developed countries; and
  - over several decades, the prevalence of diabetes has increased substantially, from around 1% to over 10%.
- NCDs are also associated with an increasing economic burden, projected to reach trillions of yuan renminbi over the next few decades.
- China has developed some national strategies for preventing NCDs and it will, in future, have better involvement of its public health and primary care systems in preventive measures and will develop more rigorous regulations in order to help to stem the rise of NCDs.
- Pharmaceutical policy changes and broader health system reforms must play a role in addressing these challenges (e.g. through the availability of cheap and effective medications).

4.1 Improvements in health indicators

Health conditions in China have vastly improved since the 1990s in spite of negative changes to its health care system in the 1980s and 1990s. Average life expectancy at birth increased from 68 to 72 years between 1990 and 2007 and reached 75 years in 2010, ranking among the highest of developing countries (Fang, 2015; Wang et al., 2013). As of 2012, maternal mortality rates were 24.5 per 100 000, down from 51.3 in 2002 (Fang, 2015). Similarly, infant mortality rates have fallen from 29.2 per 1000 in 2002 to 10.3 in 2012. A recent study of provincial childhood mortality rates in China showed that some provinces had under-5 mortality rates lower than in Canada or New Zealand, highlighting just how far parts of China have come in improving health care outcomes (Wang et al., 2015). However, there is still substantial variation in provincial life expectancy, with a 12-year spread between lowest and highest life expectancies and with those provinces with higher incomes generally faring better (Fig. 4.1) (National Bureau of Statistics of China, 2015).

Fig. 4.1 Life expectancy by province per capita GDP, 2010

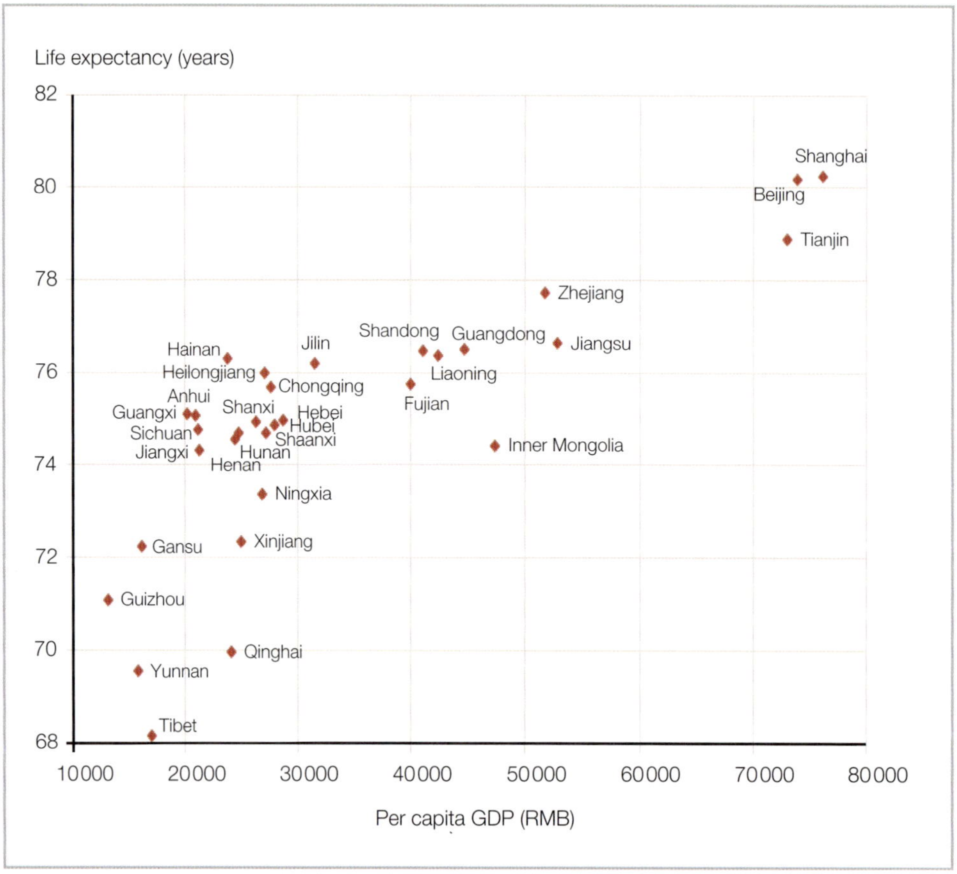

Source: National Bureau of Statistics of China, 2015.

In spite of major gains in key health outcomes, China is facing several significant issues that are fuelling an increase in the burden of NCDs: an ageing population, rapid urbanization leading to a large population of migrant workers who have difficulties accessing health care as well as significant environmental degradation and rapid lifestyle changes. China's health care system, including its pharmaceutical policies, must adapt to the needs posed by this rapid demographic and epidemiological transition.

4.2 Ageing in China

China's population is ageing rapidly. In absolute terms, China has the largest elderly population of any country in the world (Fig. 4.2) (United Nations, 2015). The proportion of the population aged 65 years or older is also projected to further increase over the next several decades (Fig. 4.3) (United Nations, 2015). The rate of ageing in China exceeds that of the rest of the world: According to a United Nations report, the global population over 60 years increased from 600 million to 841 million between 2000 to 2013, corresponding to 10% and 11% of the population, respectively (United Nations, 2013). During the same time, China's population aged over 60 increased from 129 million to 160 million, corresponding to 10% and 12% of China's total population, respectively (Wang et al., 2013). By 2050, 22% of the world's population will be over 60, compared with nearly 30% in China (United Nations, 2013).

Although an ageing population is indicative of social development and improved health conditions, it costs significantly more to care for the elderly. Any approach to reforming a health care system must take into consideration this significant demographic change.

Fig. 4.2 Selected country populations aged 65 and over, 2015 and projected for 2050

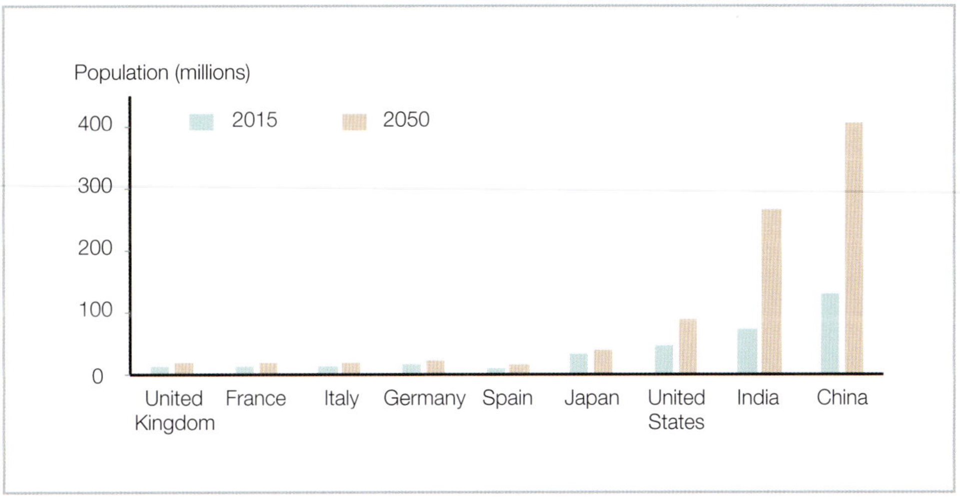

Source: National Bureau of Statistics of China, 2015.

Fig. 4.3 Proportion of China's population aged 65 and over, 1990–2015 and projected to 2050

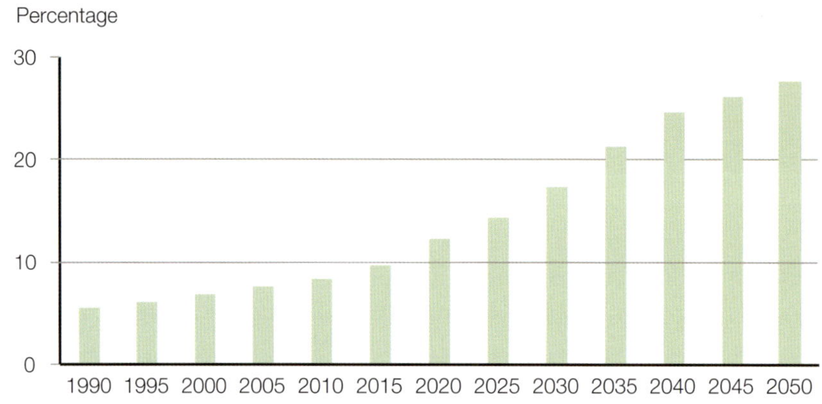

Source: United Nations, 2015.

4.3 Urbanization

China's substantial economic reforms and industrialization since the 1980s have resulted in extensive urbanization (Mattke et al., 2014; Wang et al., 2013). China has undergone the largest and most rapid human migration in history (Gong et al., 2012). The urban population increased from 191 million to 622 million between 1980 and 2009, with an additional 200 million rural-to-urban migrants expected by 2020 (Gong et al., 2012; Yusuf & Saich, 2008). By 2050, the world urban population is expected to increase by 2.5 billion, of which 292 million (12%) is expected to be in China (United Nations, 2014). In fact, China and India together will contribute to over one third of the world's projected urban population growth through to the year 2050 (United Nations, 2014). As of 2011, 51.3% of the Chinese population lived in urban areas.

Since 1990, migration movement trends have predominantly been from inland China towards the southeastern coastal provinces, where major centres of industrial growth are located. In particular, the provinces of Guangdong and Zhejiang have experienced the most net migration, accounting for approximately 38% of total interprovince migration since 1995 (Chan, 2012). China has several heavily populated regions at present, and continued internal migration will lead to more. The United Nations defines "megacities" as those with at least 10 million inhabitants and China has 6 of the world's 28 megacities plus 10 large cities with populations between 5 and 10 million (United Nations, 2014). By 2030, China is projected to have a further megacity and six more large cities, likely in the southeastern coastal regions. In early 2016, the five largest cities by population are Shanghai, Beijing, Tianjin, Guangzhou and Shenzhen (World Population Review, 2016).

This urbanization has significant implications for health. Health benefits stemming from better access to health services, higher incomes and education will likely continue to accrue to urban rather than rural residents (Box 4.1). However, consideration must also be given to the difficulties associated with health service delivery to rural migrants in urban locations; the growing disease burden in urban regions, attributable to the changing behaviours associated with an urban lifestyle; and high levels of pollution.

Box 4.1 China's rural–urban divide

Disparities in health outcomes

There are considerable differences between the health of the rural and urban populations. For example, in 2010, newborn mortality, infant mortality and under-5 mortality were all higher in rural areas (Wang et al., 2013). Rural residents are also more likely to have chronic health problems such as cancer, heart disease and arthritis and have generally poorer health status than their urban counterparts (Chen, Yin & Xie, 2014).

Disparities in health care services

In 2006, the number of doctors per 1000 people in urban and rural areas were 2.26 and 1.05, respectively. The disparity in nurses was even worse, with 1.74 and 0.53 per 1000 people in urban and rural areas, respectively (Wang et al., 2013). The number of rural practitioners has gradually increased, but numbers are still significantly lower than urban averages. In addition, the quality of health care services in rural areas is significantly lower than that in urban areas, as most health care practitioners have had far less training than their urban counterparts (Chen, Yin & Xie, 2014).

Improvements in health disparities

While gaps persist in these indicators, they have been narrowing over the past several years. One example where China has closed the rural–urban gap has been with maternal mortality. The maternal mortality rate in rural areas was two to three times higher than in urban areas between 1995 and 2005 but by 2010 parity had been reached (Chen, Yin & Xie, 2014). Similarly, in 1993 hepatitis B vaccination rates were less than 50% in rural areas compared with 90% in urban areas. By 2006, this gap had narrowed with vaccination rates of over 80% in most rural areas compared with 95% in urban areas (Gong et al., 2012).

In 2003, 55% and 21%, respectively, of urban and rural residents had health insurance. However, by 2011 coverage increased to 89% and 97.5%, respectively, with rural residents surpassing urban residents in coverage (Chen, 2012). Between 2003 and 2011, the gap between the lowest and highest income quartiles also decreased for a number of health indicators (Meng et al., 2012). The expansion of NCMS seems to have been instrumental in narrowing the inequalities in access between rural and urban areas (Meng et al., 2012). Even so, the amount of coverage offered by NCMS is far less than the urban schemes.

4.4 Migrant workers

The massive rural-to-urban migration has created unique challenges for health care delivery among the highly mobile and often undocumented migrant worker population. Many issues are also exacerbated by the fact that migrants as well as their children tend to significantly underuse health services in cities they work in and in their rural hometowns (Gong et al., 2012). A study based in Shenzhen, a popular destination in China for migrants, showed that 62% of its migrant working population who reported an illness did not visit a physician and that 55% of them were uninsured (Mou et al., 2009). Immunization rates for children of migrant workers are much lower than those for both their urban and rural counterparts (Gong et al., 2012). Reasons for the low immunization rates include lack of awareness of immunization among migrant parents, the costs associated with vaccines, frequent job-related changes of residence and births that violated the one-child policy (Gong et al., 2012). Mental health is another area where migrant workers face unique challenges linked to the stress of work, separation from families and stigma in new cities. Studies have demonstrated significantly worse mental health among migrant workers than in their city-born peers (Mou et al., 2013).

China's previous attempts to address these issues have mainly involved establishing more CHCs in popular urban migrant destinations. For example, in 2006, Beijing began offering free diagnosis and treatment for tuberculosis and HIV/AIDS in their CHCs. Children of migrant workers were also provided with health care services equal to those of registered urbanites (Gong et al., 2012). In 2010, there was a pilot project that aimed to provide health services and education for migrant workers in 65 major cities across 29 provinces (Gong et al., 2012). Unfortunately, these services are underused by migrant workers. There is also a fear that infected migrant workers, who often go undiagnosed and untreated, will increase the morbidity burden in urban areas and risk reintroduction of previously controlled diseases (Yi-Xin & Manderson, 2005). Indeed, there is some evidence that migrant workers have increased the spread of multidrug-resistant tuberculosis in urban centres (Mou et al., 2013). Tackling the health challenges faced by China's large migrant worker population and their families is a crucial task of the overall health reform.

4.5 Environmental problems

Problems with water and air quality pose significant health risks in China. Rapidly growing urban populations are putting tremendous strain on municipal water suppliers. In 2006, a survey of water suppliers revealed that more than one quarter of public water plants and more than half of private plants were not complying with monitoring requirements for water quality (Gong et al., 2012). It is feared that further migration to cities will place more pressure on suppliers to the point where they may risk tapping contaminated water sources to meet public demand (Zhang et al., 2010).

Similarly, rapid urbanization has harmed air quality. Vast increases in the number of motor vehicles and in household energy consumption, and continued coal burning, are increasing air pollution to very hazardous levels (Gong et al., 2012; World Bank & State Environmental Protection Administration, 2007). According to the World Bank, air pollution caused 400 000 premature deaths in China in 2007 (World Bank & State Environmental Protection Administration, 2007). A more recent 2015 paper from Berkeley Earth estimated that air pollution was responsible for 1.6 million premature deaths (Rohde & Muller, 2015). Stories about poor air quality are common in the popular media, with one particularly bad pollution day in Beijing (levels of particulate matter $PM_{2.5}$ pollutant were 25 times higher than safe recommended levels) reported widely as an "airpocalypse" (Lim, 2014).

4.6 NCDs

4.6.1 Lifestyle changes and NCDs

Dramatic lifestyle changes linked to urbanization have led to an epidemic of NCDs in China (Mattke et al., 2014; Wang et al., 2005; Wang et al., 2013). The underlying reason for this is that urban environments promote behaviours and lifestyles that exacerbate hypertension, high cholesterol and blood glucose levels and obesity, which are strong risk factors for diseases such as diabetes, cardiovascular diseases and cancer. Unhealthy diets, lack of activity and high smoking rates are the primary lifestyle risk factors for NCDs in China. Indeed, in 2010, 580 million Chinese were estimated to have at least one NCD risk factor (Fig. 4.4) (World Bank, 2011).

Fig. 4.4 Prevalence of risk factors for NCDs in China, 2010

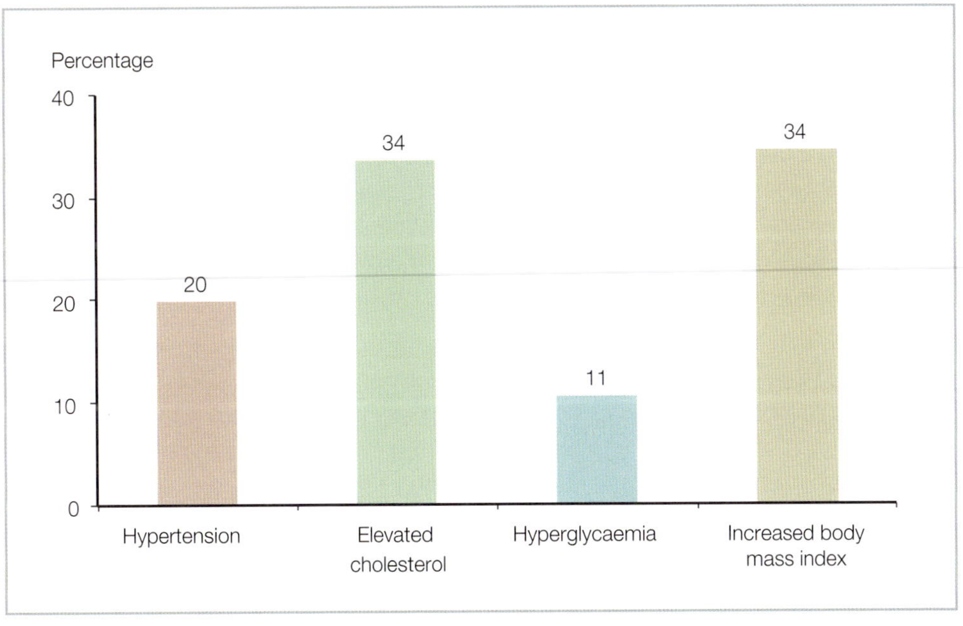

Source: World Bank, 2011.

Since the 1980s, there has been a major change in the Chinese diet. The traditional diet contained only 15% total fat and negligible amounts of sugar (Mattke et al., 2014). However, owing to changes in food supply from improved agricultural production and increased imports, the average fat content of the Chinese diet increased from 25% to 35% in urban regions and from 14% to 28% in rural areas between 1982 and 2002 (Mattke et al., 2014). Sugar intake has also increased from greater consumption of fructose-sweetened soft drinks (World Bank, 2011). Both fat and sugar intake are higher than WHO recommended levels. At the same time, average exercise levels have decreased. Less than 33% of the Chinese population reported exercising more than three times per week (Wang et al., 2013) and 16% of the population reported reduced activity levels owing to improved infrastructure and public transportation coupled with longer workdays (Wang et al., 2013). A discussion on increasing obesity rates, one of the results of these lifestyle changes, is presented in Box 4.2. Furthermore, smoking rates in China are very high, particularly among men (Box 4.3).

Box 4.2 Obesity in China

Obesity is a risk factor for a number of conditions, including diabetes, cardiovascular diseases, respiratory disease and numerous cancers. The WHO estimates that it accounts for 2.3% of all global disability-adjusted life years (WHO, 2015a). Obesity rates have increased at alarmingly fast rates in the decades since market liberalization. Between 1992 and 2002, the prevalence of overweight and obese individuals in China increased by 38% and 81%, respectively, to reach 22.8% and 7.1%, respectively (World Bank, 2011). Amongst those aged 7 to 18 years, overweight/obesity rates were 17.6% in wealthy northern coastal cities and were 32.5% in boys. A more recent study looking at data from 2004 to 2010 demonstrated a total increase in mean body mass index among all Chinese adults from 22.7 to 23.7 (Jiang et al., 2015). Central obesity, another marker of poor health status, reached 32.3% by 2010. A recent meta-analysis of children and adolescents found an increase in overweight or obesity from 1.8% and 0.4%, respectively, in 1981–1985 to 13.1% and 7.5%, respectively, in 2006–2010 (Yu et al., 2012). Different studies use different measures for estimation of overweight and obesity as there is some evidence that poor health outcomes occur at lower body mass index values among Chinese. Regardless of the body mass index value used as the cut-off or the variations in methodologies, all the evidence points towards drastic increases in obesity.

China's obesity problem is reflective of a broader global trend. Much of the developed world has reached the energy balance "flipping point", which is marked by an net increase in caloric intake due to falling levels of physical activity as well as easy access to energy-rich foods (Swinburn et al., 2011). Increasing urbanization and use of motor vehicles (large cities are no longer clogged with bicycles as they once were but rather with cars), decreasing manual labour and easy access to sugar-rich and fat-rich foods have been instrumental in driving up obesity rates in China. Certain cultural factors also contribute: within China, fatness is a sign of happiness and abundance and children are overfed by family members, particularly within the

(continued)

Box 4.2 Obesity in China (continued)

context of a one-child system (Wang & Zhai, 2013). One study even reported that children who were primarily looked after by their grandparents rather than parents were more likely to be overweight (Li, Adab & Cheng, 2015). China's obesity problem is not spread equally among the population but rather reflects a socioeconomic gradient where those who are wealthier, more politically connected and live in cities are more likely to be overweight/obese than those who are not (He et al., 2014).

As with other chronic diseases, obesity is associated with high direct and indirect costs. A systematic review of the direct costs of obesity estimated that it accounts for 0.7–2.8% of a country's THE, and that individuals who were obese had medical costs 30% higher than those who were normal weight (Withrow & Alter, 2011). A Chinese study estimated that overweight and obesity amounted to RMB91 billion, or about 4.5% of THE in 2010 (Zhang, Shi & Liang, 2013).

China has introduced a number of strategies to combat obesity (Wang & Zhai, 2013). In 2003, the Ministry of Health introduced guidelines for the prevention and control of overweight and obesity of Chinese adults. In 2007, a similar document was issued for school-age children and teenagers. Nutrition guidelines and physical activity guidelines were released in 2008 and 2010, respectively. Targeting schools is a priority as well, given the increasing rates of childhood obesity and the environmental and social opportunities available at schools to promote healthy lifestyles. Nevertheless, the majority of the government's initiatives have been in the area of health education and evaluation evidence is limited. There has been little regulatory control such as marketing restrictions, food labelling laws or taxes on unhealthy products. In the future, a more coordinated and systematic approach will be needed to stem the increasing rates of obesity in China.

Box 4.3 Smoking in China

China is home to a third of the world's 1 billion smokers and millions die every year from tobacco-related diseases such as cancer, heart attacks and stroke. Experts estimate that if smoking rates are not reduced, 100 million Chinese will die over the next century from smoking (The Economist, 2014a). In spite of the obvious health ramifications, tobacco control in China is a challenging business as the agency in charge of tobacco production, the State Tobacco Monopoly Administration, generates about 7% of yearly central government revenue and enjoys patronage at a senior level (Li, 2012). Substantive reforms that decrease smoking, such as significantly higher taxes on cigarettes, smoking bans and tobacco advertising moratoriums, will require significant support from policy-makers at the top of government.

In 2010 a large survey indicated that 28% of Chinese smoked (53% of men and only 2% of women), a rate far higher than in almost every OECD country. The health consequences of this are devastating: 1.2 million die every year from smoking-related causes, out of which 100 000 deaths are from second-hand smoke. The WHO estimates that if these trends continue, the number of tobacco-related deaths in China will increase to 3 million a year by 2050 (WHO, 2015b). Similar numbers were predicted in a recent study published in the Lancet, a prestigious medical journal. This study estimated that, in the decade from 2010 to 2020, smoking would be directly responsible for 20% of all adult male deaths in China, with an attributable mortality that would only increase with time barring major corrective efforts (Chen et al., 2015).

One of the reasons tobacco control in China is so difficult is that the industry generates substantial tax revenues. The State Tobacco Monopoly Administration has control over the world's largest tobacco firm, a conglomerate that oversees 33 province-level tobacco bureaus and 19 major tobacco companies and produces 40% of the world's cigarettes. Since the early 2000s, the State Tobacco Monopoly Administration has consistently contributed 7–10% of annual central government revenues; in 2012 this was equal to RMB 865 billion (Li, 2012). Unlike in developed countries where tobacco revenues are stagnant, the profits increased by about 20% every year from 2006 to 2010. The Chinese Academy of Social Sciences also estimates that over 60 million people are in part employed by the tobacco industry. In spite of the size of the tobacco economy, smoking creates significant direct and indirect medical costs. A 2010 study suggested that total tobacco-related costs were RMB 184 billion in 2008 (Yang et al., 2011). As more advanced medicines to treat smoking-related illness become more widespread, health care costs are sure to increase.

China's top leadership has come a long way from Deng Xiaoping, who famously smoked two packs a day and was frequently photographed with a cigarette in hand. As of December 2013, leaders have been banned from smoking in public and from using public funds to buy cigarettes. However, the brother of China's Premier Li Keqiang was until very recently the deputy director of the State Tobacco Monopoly Administration while Peng Liyuan, the wife of President Xi Jinping, has served as an "Anti-Smoking Ambassador" for the Chinese Association on Tobacco Control since 2009 (Li, 2012). All this makes for an interesting milieu for tobacco control at the highest political levels.

(continued)

Box 4.3 Smoking in China (continued)

Misperceptions also abound among average Chinese about the effects of tobacco. A 2014 WHO report demonstrated that only half of Chinese believed that smoking causes heart attacks and only a quarter believed it causes strokes – two conditions that are leading causes of death and disability in China. In fact, a 2008 survey revealed that only about 40% of physicians felt that smoking should be banned in bars (WHO, 2014b).

In spite of the many challenges to tobacco control in China, there have been various high-level and grassroots efforts to curb tobacco usage in China. A landmark achievement was China's signing of the WHO Framework Convention on Tobacco Control in 2003, a legally binding convention that has been ratified by 178 countries and stipulates a comprehensive series of measures aimed at reducing both demand and supply for cigarettes, such as heavy taxes and a total ban on tobacco advertising. Since then there have been various measures to curb smoking, such as the "Smoke-free Beijing Olympics" initiative, the introduction of basic text warnings on cigarette packaging in 2009, and a 2011 Ministry of Health ban on smoking in 28 types of public venue such as hotels, restaurants and public transit (unfortunately, enforcement remains weak). Recently, Beijing appears to have successfully banned indoors smoking, an optimistic development.

Ultimately, if China is to decrease smoking rates it will have to address a number of issues directly. The most pressing is to wean itself from the revenues from cigarette sales. Heavier taxes on cigarettes may help to sustain revenue while cutting usage. The government will need to better enforce its edicts on smoking bans and tobacco advertisements. More provocative labelling of cigarette packages, including graphic colour depictions of disease, is a well-tested method of deterring smokers. Finally, the populace needs to be better educated about just how bad smoking truly is for health, as too many do not understand the strong causal link between smoking and heart disease, stroke and cancer.

China is undergoing an epidemiological transition marked by decreasing infectious diseases and increasing NCDs. A subanalysis of the Global Burden of Disease Study examined the leading causes of years of life lost across time in China; in 1990, lower respiratory infections and preterm birth complications were the leading cause of years of life lost in half of China's provinces but by 2013 the leading causes in all provinces were cerebrovascular disease, ischaemic heart disease or lung cancer (Zhou M et al., 2015). Three of four of the leading causes of death were NCDs: cardiovascular diseases, cancer and chronic respiratory disease (Fig. 4.5) (WHO, 2014a). The WHO predicts that more than 100 million Chinese individuals will die from an NCD between 2010 and 2030 (Mattke et al., 2014). The rapid increase in diabetes prevalence has been particularly problematic in China (Box 4.4).

Fig. 4.5 Causes of mortality in China, 2014

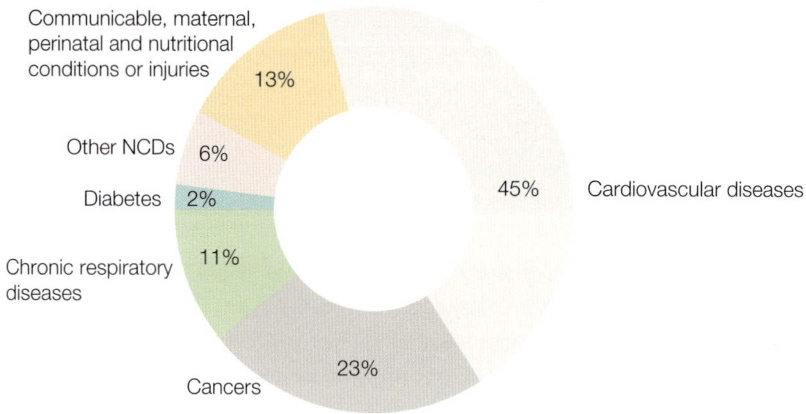

Source: WHO, 2014a.

Box 4.4 Diabetes in China

Diabetes has become one of the most challenging health problems in China. Prevalence has grown at explosive rates over a short period of time. In 1994, a national survey of over 200 000 Chinese residents found that the prevalences of diabetes and impaired glucose tolerance were 2.5% and 3.2%, respectively (Pan et al., 1997). These numbers were approximately three times greater than those reported in 1980 (Yang W et al., 2010). A study in 2000 of a nationally representative sample of over 15 000 adults reported that the prevalence of diabetes and impaired fasting glucose were 5.5% and 7.3%, respectively (Gu et al., 2003).

In 2010 another large and nationally representative study of 46 239 adults was conducted. Overall, 9.7% of the adult population (equivalent to 92.4 million adults) was found to have diabetes (Yang W et al., 2010). Furthermore, in 60.7% of these, the diabetes was undiagnosed, which meant that these patients were not seeking medical treatment for their condition. In addition, 15.5% (148.2 million adults) had pre-diabetes, which is a significant risk factor for the development of full-blown diabetes and cardiovascular diseases. Globally, approximately 50–80% of patients with diabetes eventually die from cardiovascular diseases, stroke, kidney failure and other diabetes-related complications (Jia, 2014). The growth in diabetes prevalence, fuelled by urbanization and changing lifestyles, has been remarkable.

As with other NCDs, diabetes is associated with tremendous economic costs. In 2010, the direct costs alone of treating diabetes were RMB 159 billion, a figure projected to increase to RMB 286 billion by 2030 (Wang et al., 2009). Furthermore, it has been estimated that 29% of global diabetes treatment between 2015 and 2025 will take place in China (Alcorn & Ouyang, 2012). Given its substantial health and economic burden, national strategies and policies should prioritize the effective prevention, detection and treatment of diabetes for all Chinese.

The economic costs associated with NCDs in China is very high. NCDs are the largest contributor to increasing health expenditure. For example, between 1985 and 2005, health expenditure associated with cardiovascular diseases increased by 17.3% annually, far higher than the 11.8% annual increase in THE (World Bank, 2011). One study estimated the costs associated with the five largest NCDs (cardiovascular diseases, cancer, chronic respiratory disease, diabetes and mental health) between 2010 and 2030 will be an enormous RMB 177 trillion (Bloom et al., 2013).

4.6.2 Dealing with NCDs

As part of its 12th Five Year Plan, the Chinese Government committed to a National Plan for NCD Prevention between 2012 and 2015, which focused on prevention, surveillance, supportive social environments and primary health care (China CDC, 2012). The plan includes a list of goals to be reached by 2015, some of which include:

- reduce mean daily salt intake to <9 g;
- reduce adult smoking rate to <25%;
- increase the proportion of population that exercises regularly to >32%;
- reduce obesity rates to <12% of adults and <8% of children/teenagers;
- reduce rates of chronic obstructive pulmonary disease in adults to <8%; and
- ensure that 40% of hypertensive and diabetic patients are able to manage their disease, with 60% of diabetics being able to adequately control their blood sugar levels.

The key strategies to reach these goals include using mass media methods to raise awareness for NCD prevention, providing guidance for healthy diets, implementing the general principles for nutrition labelling of prepackaged foods, ensuring that primary and secondary students participate in one hour of physical exercise during school days, instituting a smoking ban in public places and improving NCD surveillance.

While having a national strategy for NCD prevention is a good starting point, China will need to reorient much of its health system in order to combat NCDs. Public health could play a much larger role in helping to prevent NCDs through education and outreach activities and by playing a role in addressing upstream determinants of NCDs, including ensuring people live in healthy built environments. A stronger primary care system would enable earlier detection and treatment of disease as well as better case management of those with advanced NCDs. Regulation is also important: China has so far been quite weak at limiting the power of tobacco manufacturers and has little in the way of advertising limits or taxes on unhealthy foods.

4.7 Conclusions

While China has made impressive gains in health outcomes over the past several decades, moving forwards it is facing a unique and substantial set of health care challenges. A rapidly ageing population, rapid urbanization and changes in lifestyle have fuelled a rapid rise in NCDs that have severe health consequences for the Chinese people. In the 1980s, infections were the leading cause of death and disability in China but now the leading causes are all NCDs, such as cardiovascular diseases, cancer and chronic respiratory disease. China has one of the world's highest smoking rates, diabetes rates that have exploded in the past few decades and increasing levels of obesity among adults and children.

China needs a coordinated strategy for dealing with NCDs. The 12th Five Year Plan sets ambitious targets for NCD prevention but requires actions by public health and primary care backed by strong regulations to reach its goals. The economic burden of treating NCDs is already quite high and is only projected to increase. Consequently, preventing their increase is all the more important, both to ensure the health of Chinese and to help to contain what could be exorbitantly high health care costs.

Many NCDs such as hypertension, diabetes, cardiovascular diseases and cancer require pharmacological treatment for optimal management. As a result, pharmaceutical policy will play an important role in their management. Policies that promote accessible and affordable medications for common NCDs throughout urban and rural areas will be essential. This can be done by promoting the broad use of high-quality, low-cost generic medications as many of the key drugs to treat NCDs are off-patent. Standardized clinical pathways for common NCDs will also help to ensure rational use of medications so that the best clinical outcome is obtained for the lowest cost.

5. Trends in health care and pharmaceutical spending

KEY MESSAGES

- Demand for health care use is rising rapidly and is largely centred on an increased number of hospital as well as inpatient visits.
- Health spending is growing rapidly, with an annual rate of over 15% over recent years. However, spending as percentage of GDP is only 5.4%, far below the OECD average.
- There is wide geographic variation in spending, with wealthier provinces spending up to three times per capita what poorer provinces spend.
- OOP expenditure is gradually decreasing as government expenditure is increasing. However, it still makes up more than a third of THE and up to 10% of the total disposable income of rural residents.
- Pharmaceutical spending constitutes over 35% of THE and has been decreasing gradually as a share of THE. Growth in pharmaceutical spending has been very high in past years but is set to slow quite dramatically in the coming years.
- Within hospitals, pharmaceutical spending is almost equally split between inpatient and outpatient care. Drug expenses make up 40–50% of both inpatient and outpatient visit costs and are increasing for outpatient visits.
- Most pharmaceutical spending is on off-patent medications, although over the next few years spending on both in-patent drugs and drugs on the EDL is projected to increase as the value of off-patent originators falls.

5.1 Increasing demand for health care in China

Demand for health care is rising in China. From 2005 to 2012, the total number of visits to all health care institutions grew by 68%, from 4.1 to 6.9 billion visits. The use of inpatient services grew by 148% over this period, from 71.2 to 178.1 million visits. Hospital demand grew more than the use of primary care facilities, from 1.4 billion to 2.5 billion (83%) compared with 2.6 billion to 4.1 billion visits (58%) for primary care (Center for Health Statistics and Information, 2013). Inpatient visits grew by 148% over that period, compared with only 67% for outpatient visits.

5.2 Trends in THE

China's THE has been growing quickly and steadily. From 2005 to 2012, THE grew from RMB 866 billion to RMB 2812 billion. As a percentage of total GDP, THE increased from 4.68% to 5.36% during this period. While growth in THE has been fast, THE as a percentage of GDP is still far lower than the 2012 OECD average of 9.3%, while it is in the mid range of those seen in the five major emerging national economies: Brazil (10%), Russia (7%), India (4%), China (5.5%) and South Africa (9%) (the BRICS countries; OECD, 2014; WHO, 2014c). Health care spending in China is calculated based on the official revenues of health care institutions rather than through incurred expenditures. As a result, some OOP payments, for example to nurses employed directly by patients, as well as any unofficial income such as "red envelopes" are not included in official figures. Consequently, official estimates are lower than true spending (Development Research Center of the State Council, 2015). The extent of the underestimation is difficult to assess.

In absolute terms, per capita THE in China was only US$ 480, seven times less the OECD average of US$ 3484 (Fig. 5.1) (OECD, 2014; WHO, 2014c). THE has been consistently outpacing GDP growth, and between 2008 and 2012, it increased at an annual rate of 14.2%. During this period, government expenditure increased most rapidly, at an average annual rate of 18.6%, compared with 14.6% for social health expenditure and 10.4% for OOP expenditure.

In 2012, THE was split fairly equally between government expenditure (30.0%), social expenditure (35.7%) and OOP expenditure (34.3%) (Figs 5.2 and 5.3) (National Health Development Research Center, 2013). In recent years, there has been a significant influx of government funds to support the health care reform efforts. Consequently, government spending as a percentage of THE increased from 17.9% in 2005 to 30.0% in 2015. OOP spending peaked in the early 2000s at almost 60% of THE but has gradually been falling since then as both government and social expenditures have increased. Even though increases in government expenditure have far outpaced increases in OOP expenditure, the initially high reliance on OOP expenditure in the pre-2009 health care reform era means that significantly more government expenditure is needed to further decrease OOP spending.

There is also significant variation in per capita health expenditure by province. For example, Beijing (considered a provincial-level jurisdiction) spent RMB 5751 per capita on health care in 2012 compared with Guizhou, a poor southern province, which only spent RMB 1378 per capita. The breakdown of spending between government expenditure, social expenditure and OOP expenditure also varies significantly between provinces. Per capita expenditure and breakdown by source for selected provinces are shown in Table 5.1 (National Health Development Research Center, 2013).

Fig. 5.1 Health expenditure per capita in China and other OECD countries, 2012 or latest available year

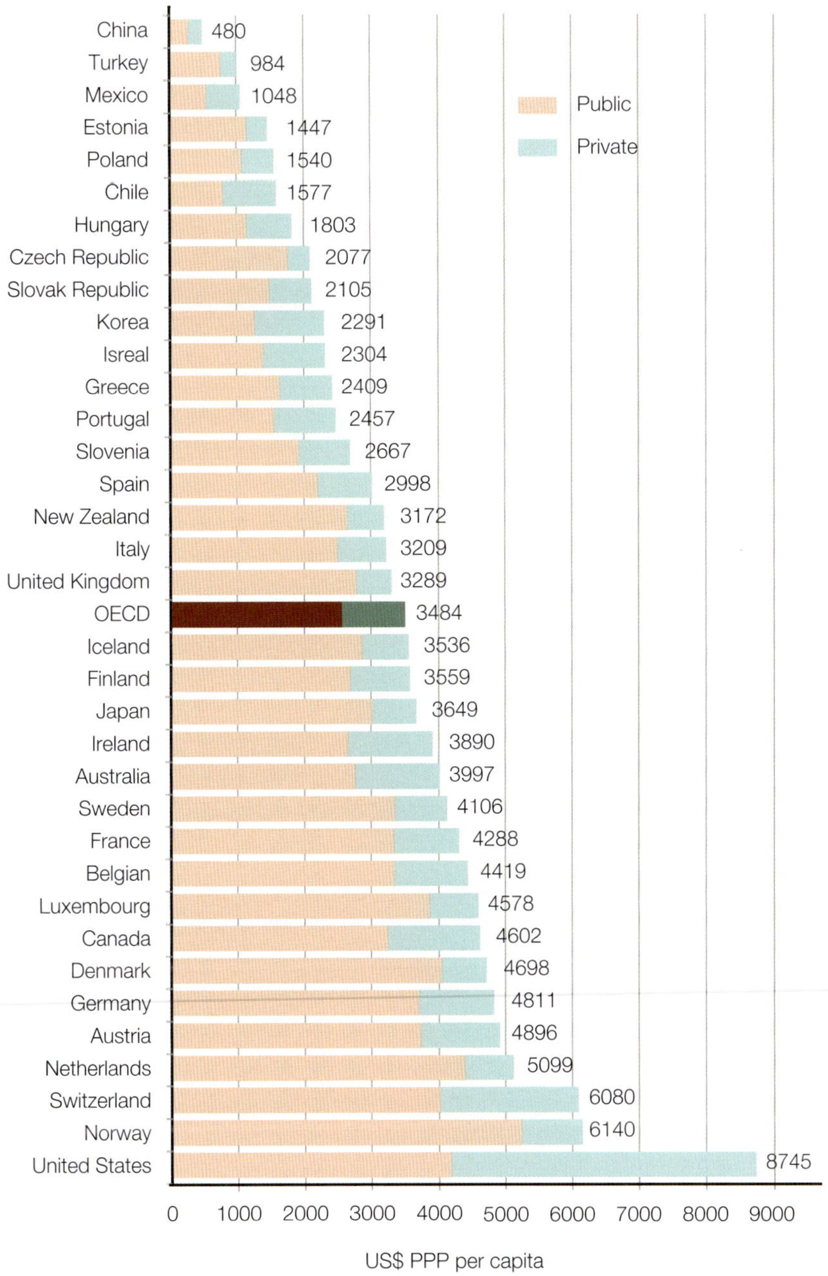

Source: OECD, 2014; WHO, 2014c.
Note: PPP: Purchasing power parity.

Fig. 5.2 Health expenditure in China by source, 1990–2012

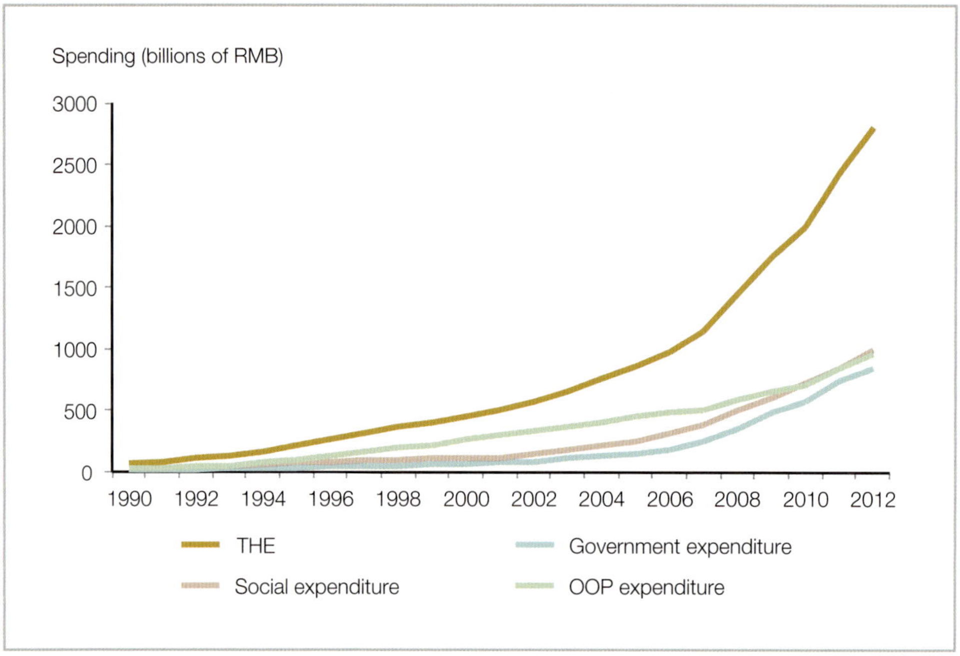

Source: National Health Development Research Center, 2013.

Fig. 5.3 Government, social and OOP expenditures as percentages of THE, 1990–2012

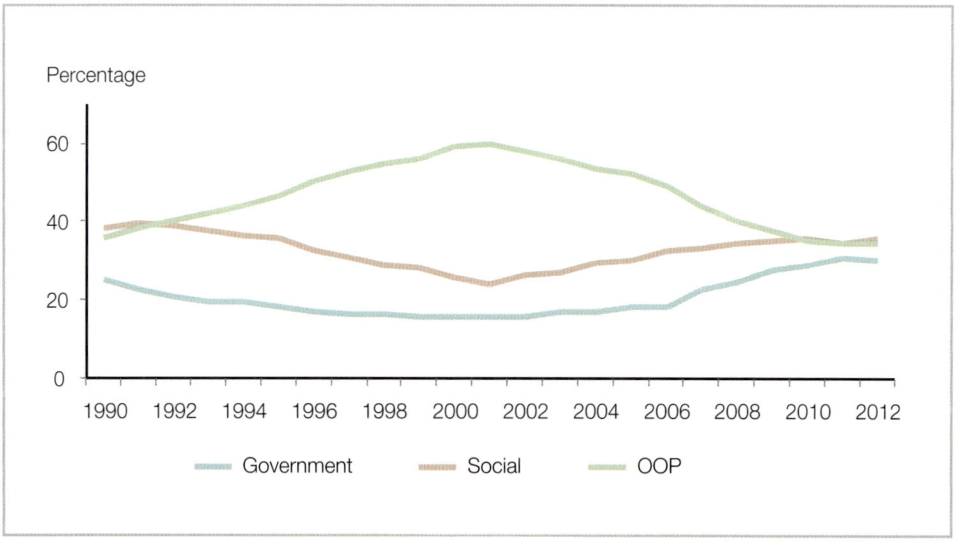

Source: National Health Development Research Center, 2013.

Table 5.1 Differences in health care spending in selected provinces, 2012

Province	Region	Per capita expenditure (RMB)	Government expenditure (%)	Social expenditure (%)	OOP expenditure (%)
Beijing	Major city	5751	26.9	50.5	22.6
Shanghai	Major city	4589	21.3	59.2	19.5
Tianjin	Major city	3394	25.2	38.4	36.4
Zhejiang	Coastal	2818	22.2	44.7	28.8
Guangdong	Coastal	2063	26.9	39.3	40.1
Heilongjiang	Northern	2148	23.2	34.0	42.3
Jilin	Northern	2356	26.9	27.4	45.7
Gansu	Western	1725	38.0	25.6	36.4
Ningxia	Western	2086	38.4	46.7	34.6
Hubei	Central	1893	28.0	30.7	41.3
Sichuan	Central	1741	33.7	33.2	33.1

Source: National Health Development Research Center, 2013.

5.3 OOP spending

OOP spending accounts for far more of THE in rural than in urban areas. In 2011, OOP spending constituted 50% of THE in rural areas, compared with only 36% in urban areas. Furthermore, OOP spending on health as a proportion of total income has actually been increasing in rural areas in spite of increased government funding in health care. As a proportion of annual income, OOP spending on health increased from 5.2 to 8.4% from 2000 to 2011 in rural areas. In the same time period in urban areas, OOP fluctuated upwards then fell again, to remain at 6.4% of annual income (Fig. 5.4) (Long et al., 2013). Higher rates of rural OOP spending is likely a reflection of higher urban incomes and more generous urban insurance schemes compared with the NCMS for rural

Fig. 5.4 OOP expenditure as a percentage of total income in rural and urban residents, 2000–2011

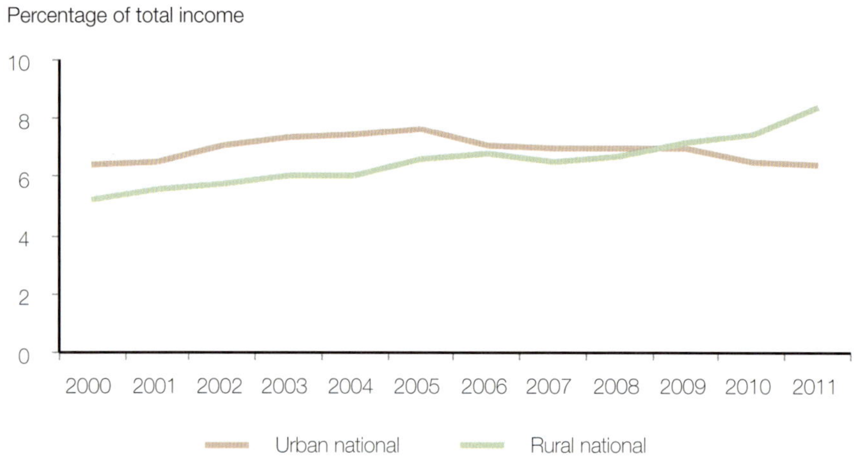

Source: Long et al., 2013.

residents (Long et al., 2013). The fact that THE accounts for 8.4% of total rural income raises serious questions about affordability.

The not insignificant rural–urban divide in OOP expenditure should be addressed by future rounds of funding that target rural residents with larger government subsidies. Unfortunately, there are no data on the percentage of OOP spending specifically on pharmaceutical products.

5.4 Pharmaceutical expenditure

China spends more on pharmaceuticals as a percentage of THE, around 40%, than the OECD average of 20% (OECD, 2015a). China's TPE:THE ratio is also higher than comparable BRICS countries, including Brazil (~12%), Russia (~18%) or India (~26%) (BMI Research, 2015; Deloitte, 2015; McKinsey, 2014; WHO, 2014c). It is well understood in China that revenue from drug sales pays for hospital operating costs and health care workers' salaries, a by-product of the 15% mark-up policy. The government has recognized the perverse incentives created from the 15% mark-up and has been trying to decrease pharmaceutical spending as a proportion of THE.

In 2012, TPE was RMB 1186 billion (per capita drug expenditure RMB 876), which represented approximately 40% of THE (Fig. 5.5) (National Health Development Research Center, 2013). From 1990 to 2009, TPE was an average of 45.7% of THE and

Fig. 5.5 TPE and THE in China, 1990–2012

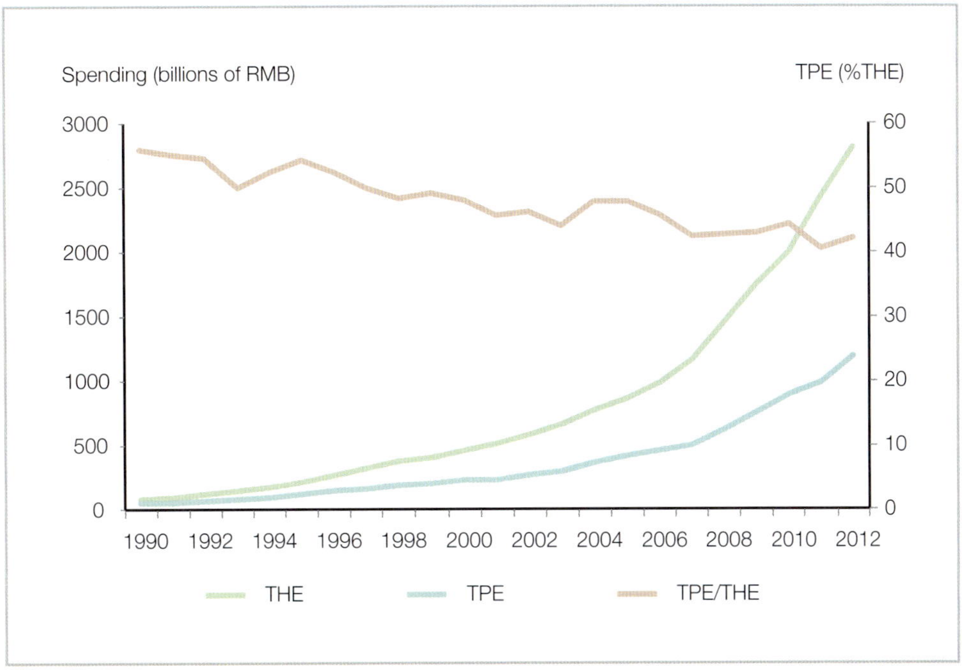

Source: National Health Development Research Center, 2013.

decreased at a rate of 0.4% per year (Shi et al., 2014). Even though TPE as a proportion of THE has gradually been falling, overall pharmaceutical spending is still growing rapidly: between 2005 and 2012, TPE increased at an average annual rate of 14.1%

OTC drug spending has also increased and as of 2011 was RMB 162 billion, representing 18% of total pharmaceutical spending (Fig. 5.6) (China Nonprescription Medicines Association, 2012). As with TPE, there has been a gradual decline in growth in OTC drug spending in recent years.

Historically, increases in overall drug spending have been driven by increases in both drug volumes (more prescribing) and drug prices (more expensive drugs). Data from a sample of selected hospitals suggest that price growth has been decreasing and that future increases in TPE will be driven by continued volume growth (IMS Health, 2014a). IMS Health, a health care consultancy, predicts that the double digit growth of the past decades is set to slow dramatically to a compound annual growth rate of 6–9% over the next five years (Fig. 5.7) (IMS Health, 2015a). Other sources project the slowdown in growth of pharmaceutical spending to persist for the next several years (CPA-McKinsey, 2015; IBISWorld, 2015c).

Fig. 5.6 Yearly spending on OTC drugs and annual growth rate, 1998–2010

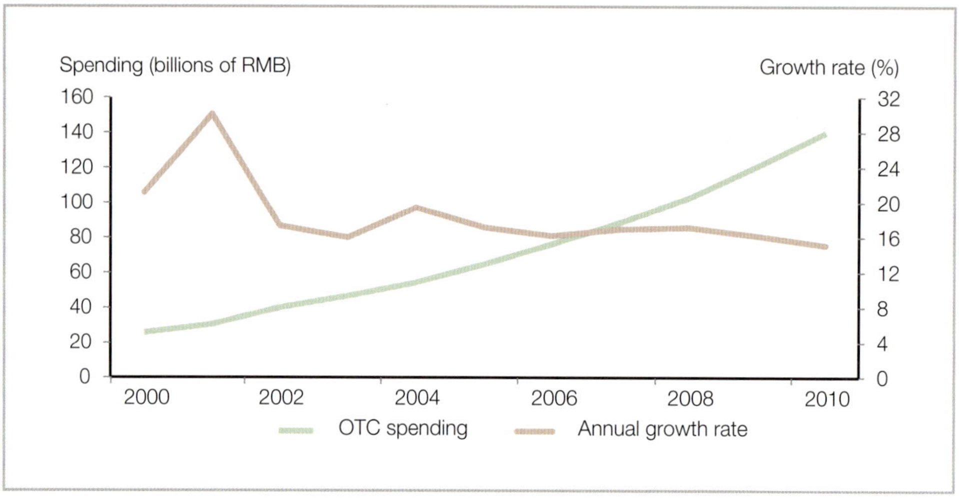

Source: China Nonprescription Medicines Association, 2012.

Fig. 5.7 Annual drug expenditure and growth rate in drug expenditure in China, 2010–2015 and forecast for 2016–2020

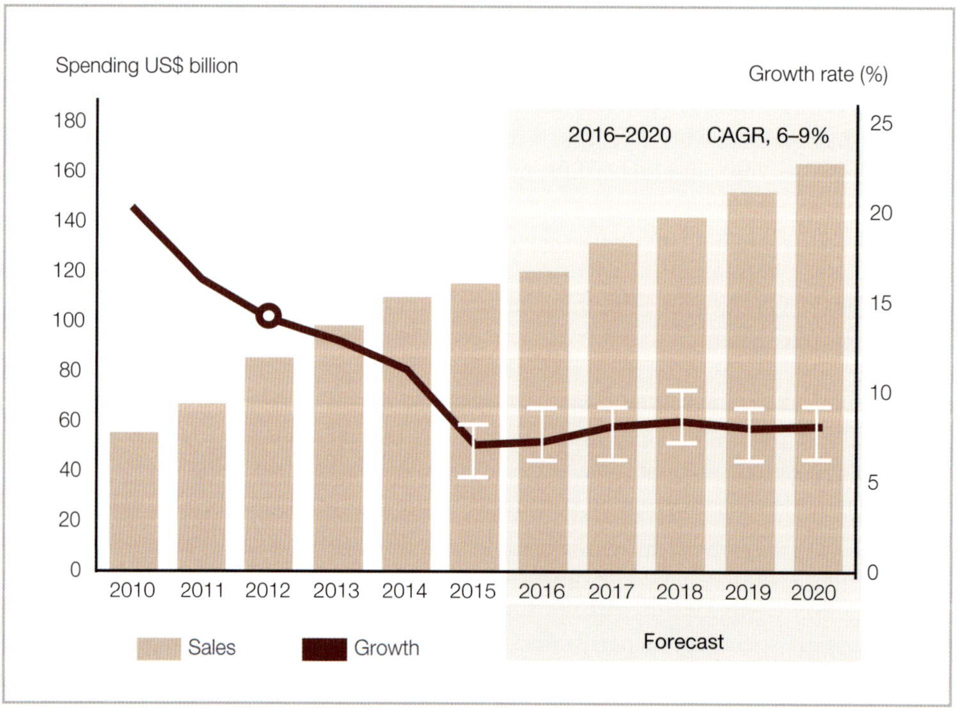

Source: IMS Health, 2015a.

Note: CAGR: Compound annual growth rate.

The majority of pharmaceutical spending occurs in hospitals and other health care institutions rather than in retail pharmacies. The proportion of drug expenditure at health care institutions was 77.8% in 2009 and gradually decreased to 73.7% in 2011 (Fig. 5.8) (Center for Health Statistics and Information, 2013). The government has been trying to encourage the use of retail pharmacies as a way to remove the link between drug sales and health care institutions. Furthermore, the high drug spending in Chinese hospitals differs from that seen in most other countries, where hospitals account for a small proportion of drug spending. For example, among a panel of OECD countries, drug spending in hospitals ranged from a low of 8% (Canada) to a high of 31% (Portugal), with most countries falling into the 10–20% range for hospital drug expenditure (OECD, 2015b).

Fig. 5.8 Breakdown of pharmaceutical spending by location, 2009–2011

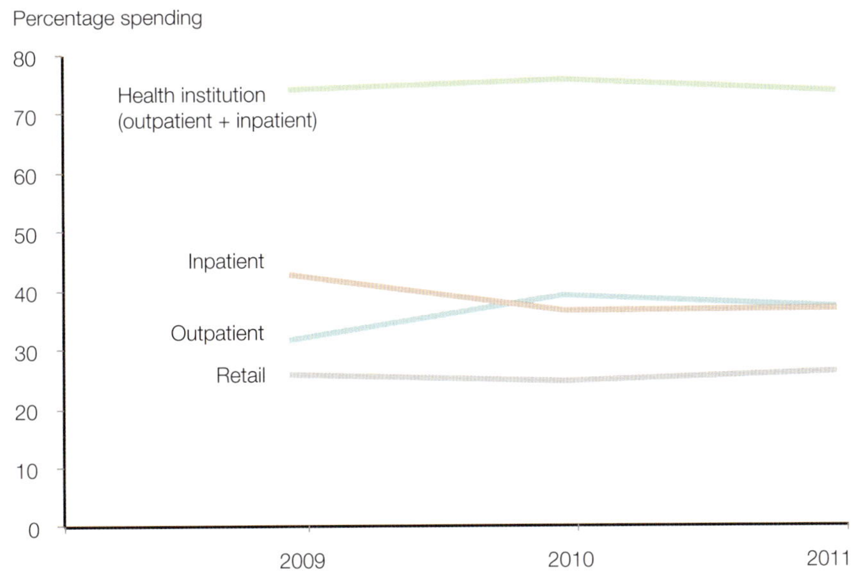

Source: Center for Health Statistics and Information, 2013.

Expenditure in health care facilities was nearly evenly divided between medications for outpatient (RMB 351 billion) and inpatient (RMB 347 billion) care. Drug costs as a percentage of total expenditure for inpatient visits decreased from 44% in 2008 to 41% in 2012 (Fig. 5.9) (Center for Health Statistics and Information, 2013). A similar trend is not seen for outpatient encounters, where drug expenditure as a percentage of total medical expenses gradually increased from 43% in 2008 to 51% in 2012. These results suggest that, at least for outpatients, the rate of growth of government subsidies and doctor and health care worker service fees (the other large component of medical expenses) was not keeping pace with the growth in drug costs.

Fig. 5.9 Drug costs as a percentage of total medical expenditure among inpatients and outpatients

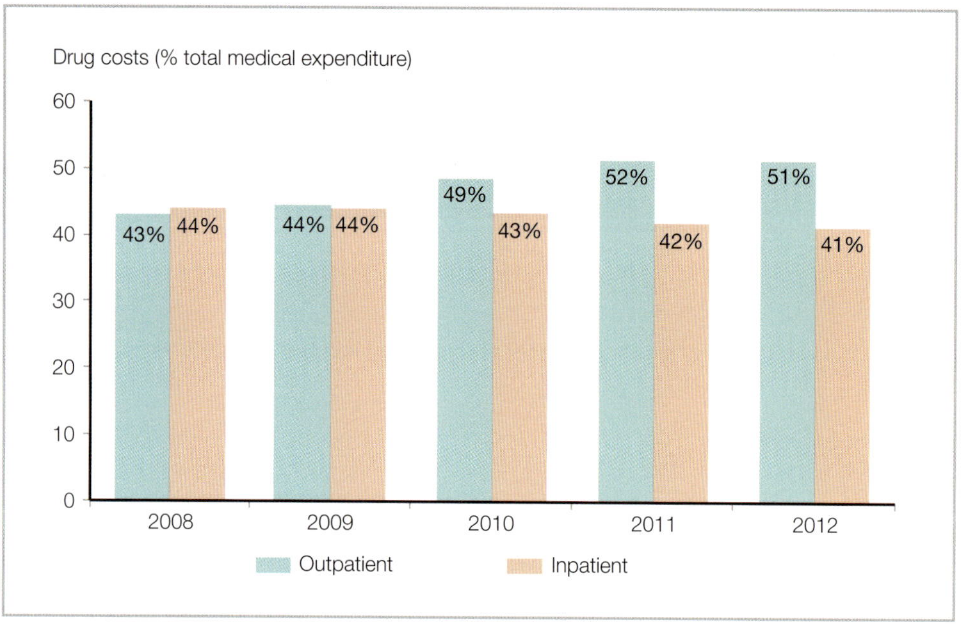

Source: Center for Health Statistics and Information, 2013.

5.5 Pharmaceutical market breakdown

Throughout the 2000s, growth in drug spending in China was the highest in the world. China has already, or will soon, overtake Japan as the country with the world's second largest pharmaceutical spend behind the United States (IMS Health, 2013d). Various consultancies have published more detailed information on the breakdown of drug spending changes.

One report projects that drug spending will increase most rapidly in county hospitals even as urban hospitals contribute the most in dollar terms to spending growth (Fig. 5.10) (Boston Consulting Group, 2014). Growth in the market is predicted to be driven by county hospitals as a result of increased incentives for patients to use county hospitals, improved infrastructure and increased number of physicians. The county hospital market is dominated by domestic pharmaceutical firms compared with cities, where multinational corporations are successful at selling patented and off-patent originator drugs. Another report, which looks at the breakdown of spending by hospital and city tier, suggests that tier 3 (the most advanced) hospitals, on the one hand, are capturing increasing market share (56% in 2009 and 65% in 2014) compared with lower tier hospitals (CPA-McKinsey, 2015). On the other hand, the overall market share of tier 1 cities (Beijing, Shanghai, Guangzhou and Shenzhen) has been decreasing (17% in 2009, 13% in 2014) as drug spending in lower tier cities accelerates.

Fig. 5.10 Growth and projected growth of pharmaceuticals by hospital category, 2008–2020[a]

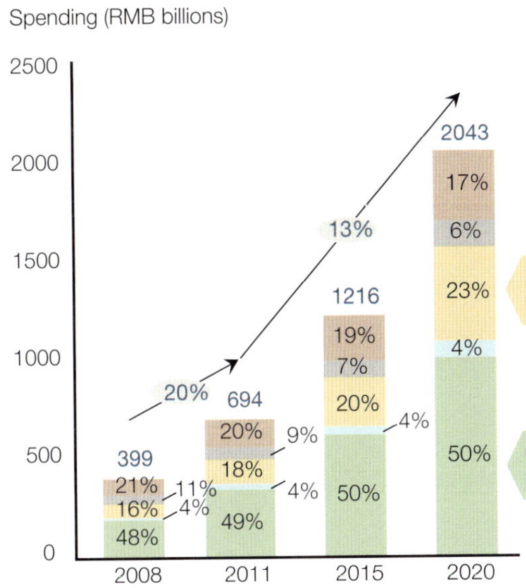

	CAGR 2008–2011 (%)	CAGR 2011–2020 (%)	Contribution to growth 2011–2020 (RMB billions)
Total	20	13	1349
Retail	19	11	215
THC	10	9	69
County hospital	24	16	352
CHC	26	12	54
City hospital	21	13	660

Source: Boston Consulting Group, 2014 (data analysed using BCG modelling from the China Health Statistic Yearbook 2012; NHFPC, Economist Intelligence Unit, and a literature search).

Notes: Based on institution purchase prices; CAGR: Compound annual growth rate.

[a] City hospitals contribute the largest absolute incremental growth but county hospitals are growing faster

Of the fastest growing classes of therapeutic drug, several are used in treating chronic diseases, with drugs used to treat diabetes, blood pressure and high cholesterol being among the top five (IMS Health, 2013a). Over the next few years, various sources project that the market for patented medications and EDL drugs will grow (Fig. 5.11) (Boston Consulting Group, 2014; IMS Health, 2015a). Growth in sales of patented drugs reflects China's increasing wealth and the expansion of public and private health insurance. Expansion of patent drugs and EDL drugs will reduce the market share of off-patent originator drugs, which many multinational corporations currently market, as well as for nondifferentiated generic drugs.

However, the total value of China's patented drug market is still far from that in developed countries. In most mature markets, patented drugs account for 60–80% of total market value while generic drugs account for the majority of total market volume (e.g. 76% in Germany, 75% in the United Kingdom and 73% in New Zealand) (OECD, 2013b).

Fig. 5.11 Breakdown of pharmaceutical share by drug type in 2011 and projections for 2020 (based on sales value but excluding the retail channel and TCM)

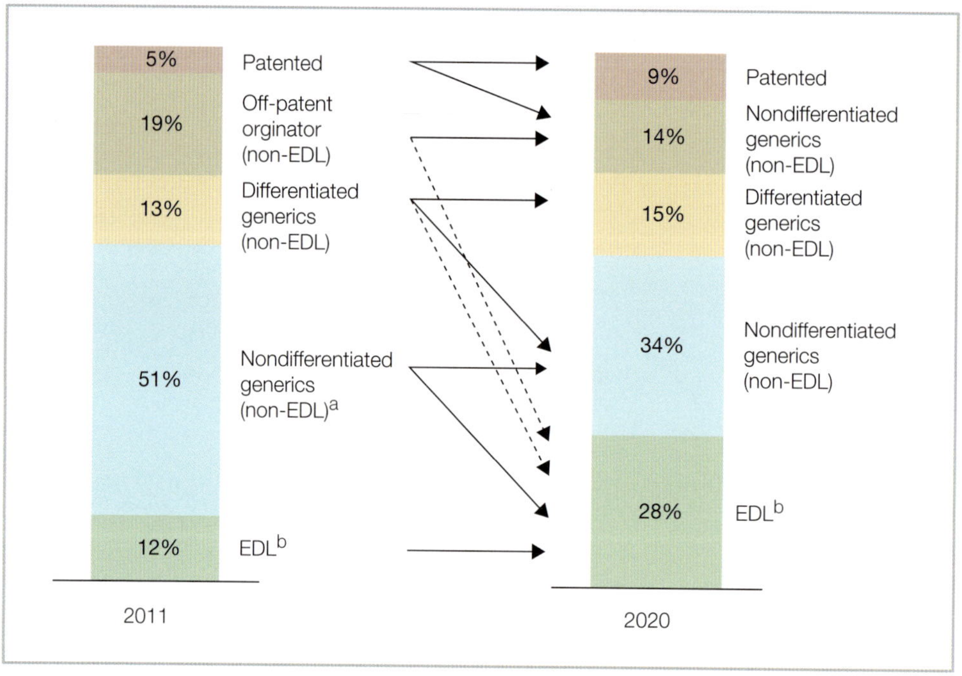

Source: Boston Consulting Group, 2014 (data analysed using BCG modelling from China Health Statistic Yearbook 2012, NHFPC, CFDA, EvaluatePharma and a literature search).

Notes: a A limited number of these drugs will move to the EDL; b EDL is mostly nondifferentiated generic drugs.

5.6 Conclusions

Health care spending in China has been growing rapidly over the past several years, particularly in light of the 2009 health care reforms. However, at 5–6% of GDP, it is still somewhat below the OECD average of around 10% of GDP. Government spending is gradually increasing while OOP expenditure is gradually decreasing, but the latter remains persistently high at about 30% of THE. Efforts to decrease OOP spending must continue to address issues of affordability and access.

Pharmaceutical spending makes up slightly less than 40% of THE. China's overall drug spending is growing rapidly and is, or soon will be, the world's second largest drug market behind the United States. Most spending still occurs in hospitals and other health care facilities, with far less at retail pharmacies. Government policies are seeking to decrease drug expenditure as a share of health spending and encourage the sale of drugs outside the hospital setting. Such policies appear to have been somewhat successful over the past few years but China is still far from OECD levels of drug spending as a percentage of GDP.

The pharmaceutical industry is projected to grow robustly, albeit at a slower rate than before. In particular, drugs that treat chronic diseases will experience the fastest growth, a reflection of their growing burden on health. There will also be a push towards lower priced generics through wider implementation of the EDL.

6. Affordability and accessibility of pharmaceuticals

KEY MESSAGES

- The 2009 health care reforms have sought to address serious problems with affordability and access in China. In spite of increased government investment through these reforms, surveys suggest the majority of Chinese still find health care to be expensive and unaffordable.
- Studies on the affordability of a basket of basic EDL and non-EDL drugs demonstrated generic prices that were relatively in line with developing county standards, but originator prices were almost ten times higher. The introduction of the EDL did not appear to lower the cost of this basket of drugs.
- In terms of accessibility, many basic medications were unavailable, and even a large percentage of EDL medications were not found at study sites in 2010. In general, availability was higher in private clinics and in higher-tier (more advanced) hospitals. Making basic medications available in primary care public facilities should be a priority.
- OOP expenditure on health as a percentage of total consumption was 6.4% for urban residents and 8.4% for rural residents. However, the figures for urban residents are declining while they appear to be increasing for rural residents. Similarly, rural households are more likely than their urban counterparts to face catastrophic health expenditures.
- While most courses of drug treatment cost less than a reference day's wages, some did not, particularly for those medications where the generic formulations are unavailable or when they are only sold at private facilities.

6.1 Health insurance in China

Broadening insurance coverage was one of the main goals of the 2009 health reforms and is a key aspect of ensuring drug access. China has three main health insurance schemes, each covering a particular demographic. The NCMS covers rural residents; the URBMI covers unemployed urban residents; and the UEBMI covers employed and retired urban residents. The NCMS and URBMI are funded through a combination of central and local government subsidies and annual individual contributions while the UEBMI is a social insurance scheme with contributions made by workers and their employers. Funds for these three insurance schemes are separate, and the UEBMI has far more resources than the NCMS or the URBMI.

Insurance coverage rates have increased to over 95% of the population in China, but there are large inequalities in the extent of coverage (Chen, 2012). Because of the different levels of funding to the three insurance schemes, what is covered, co-payment levels and reimbursement ceilings are quite different (see Table 2.1). Within the three schemes, the extent of coverage varies by region as many plans receive extra funding through local governments. These factors contribute to high OOP spending on health care and pharmaceuticals. For example, some 12.9% of Chinese households experienced catastrophic health care expenditure in 2011 (Meng et al., 2015).

China also has hundreds of millions of migrant workers who have difficulty accessing health services. In China, health care coverage and almost all other services are linked with a geographic location through a person's official registration or *hukou* (The *Wall Street Journal*, 2015). Consequently, rural workers who move to the city cannot easily access urban health insurance schemes as transference of services is challenging (Gong et al., 2012). Improving the portability of health insurance will be necessary to address the unmet needs of the migrant worker population, and deeper reforms of the hukou system are needed to address access to other services.

In the long term, increasing harmonization of the three insurance schemes is important for increasing equity of coverage. China essentially has three separate risk insurance pools, which perpetuates differences in coverage between them. There has been a move towards integrating the NCMS and the URBMI, as they have similar levels of per capita funding and are both largely tax funded, unlike the payroll-funded and much wealthier UEBMI (Development Research Center of the State Council, 2015). Incorporating the much wealthier UEBMI into the other two schemes would greatly increase the pool of resources, but there does not seem to be the appetite to do so at this juncture.

6.2 Affordability of medications

In spite of significant increases in government health care spending, there is a common perception that health care is still not affordable in China. There is a common Chinese saying that goes *kanbinggui, kanbingnan* (seeing the doctor is hard and seeing the doctor is expensive). A 2011 survey found that only 55% of Chinese felt that the 2009 reforms had improved affordability; the remainder felt there were no changes or that health care had become even more expensive (Deloitte, 2011). Another large survey conducted in 2013 showed that 95% of Chinese felt that health care was expensive and 87% felt that it was actually more expensive than four years previous when the health care reforms were launched. Finally, a survey that focused specifically on rural populations covered by the NCMS in Liaoning Province found that high drug prices were the most commonly cited reason (78.3%) for overall high medical expenses (Wang X et al., 2014b). As drug spending accounts for around 40–50% of the total cost of inpatient and outpatient visits, it contributes significantly to high medical costs (Center for Health Statistics and Information, 2013; Meng et al., 2005).

The EDL was created in part to help to control drug costs for the most basic essential medications. Four studies examined affordability and availability of medications that the authors deemed essential. The first took place in Hubei Province in 2007 using medications belonging to an older iteration of the 2009 EDL (Yang H et al., 2010). Two studies took place in Shaanxi Province in 2010 and 2012, the latter being a follow-up of the first (Jiang et al., 2013, 2014). Lastly, there was a study in Shaanxi Province that looked specifically at paediatric essential medications (Wang X et al., 2014a). The studies used WHO/Health Action International methodology to select a sample of medicines (WHO & Health Action International, 2008). Prices in the public and private sector were compared using the International Reference Price Index created by Management Sciences for Health that allows for cross-country comparisons. This gives the procurement prices for non-profit-making and profit-making suppliers to developing countries for multi-source products (Jiang et al., 2013; Yang H et al., 2010). Generally, the studies concluded that a ratio of 1 or less indicates efficient public procurement, and that ratios of less than 1.5 in the public sector and less than 2.5 in the private sector represent acceptable prices for patients. As the ratios become higher, drugs become less affordable.

Generic medicines are a specific focus, as patients with low incomes are most likely to purchase these rather than patented drugs. Particularly of interest are prices in public outlets as these are most easily affected by government price controls and reimbursements. In the public sector in 2007, the retail price for a selected sample of medicines was 1.04 times the international reference price, while in 2010 the retail price was 0.97 times the international reference price (Table 6.1) (Jiang et al., 2013, 2014; Wang X et al., 2014a; Yang H et al., 2010). This slight decrease from 2007 may represent cost-containment effects of the EDL, although regional or methodological differences could also explain the price decrease. Unfortunately, retail prices increased from 2010 to 2012 within Shaanxi Province, suggesting that after a few years the EDL was less effective at cost-containment.

Another interesting observation from these studies is the degree of mark-up between procurement and retail prices. Median mark-ups in Hubei in 2007 were 44.8%, higher than what is allowed by the 15% mark-up policy (Yang H et al., 2010). Even after the advent of the EDL and ZMU policy, mark-ups were still present in Shaanxi Province in 2010 and 2012 for both generic and off-patent originator medications at public clinics (Jiang et al. 2013, 2014). The authors suggested that the existence of a mark-up after 2009 may result from inefficiencies in the public procurement process.

Off-patent originator brands are consistently far more expensive than their generic equivalents. In 2007, their retail price was 11.25 times the international reference price in Hubei, while in 2010 in Shaanxi retail prices were 10.16 times the international reference price, rising to 11.83 times the international reference price in 2012. The existence of substantial price differences between generic drugs and off-patent originators is well known and caused in part by a perception of higher quality among originators that allows

Table 6.1 Procurement and retail prices of generics and originators in public and private clinics in relation to the international reference price

	2007 (Hubei)	2010 (Shaanxi)	2012 (Shaanxi)	2012 (Shaanxi, paediatric)
Procurement prices				
Public generics	0.74	0.75	1.49	0.52
Public off-patent originators	9.78	8.49	8.89	2.25
Retail prices				
Public generics	1.04	0.97	1.69	0.93
Private generics	0.68	1.53	1.86	1.25
Public off-patent originators	11.25	10.16	11.83	2.59
Private off-patent originators	19.94	8.36	10.72	3.89

Sources: Jiang et al., 2013, 2014; Wang X et al., 2014a; Yang H et al., 2010.

for a large price premium to be commanded. Estimates for size of these differences vary dramatically, from around 40–50% to the 1000% observed in this study (Hu et al., 2015; Zeng, 2013). Paediatric medications are generally cheaper than adult medications. Interestingly, the price gap between off-patent originators and generic medications is much less for paediatric essential medications. When patients turn to private clinics and pharmacies for their drugs, they also face much higher prices for off-patent originators. Generic drugs are also more expensive in private facilities.

The fact that the international reference price is generally close to 1 for most generics means that China's public procurement process is reasonable by global standards, at least in the sampled provinces. However, there is a huge gap between generics and off-patent originators. Finally, there were no significant price declines following the introduction of the EDL between Hubei and Shaanxi Provinces or even within Shaanxi Province between 2010 and 2012.

6.3 Health care and medication costs as a proportion of income

High OOP payments are a significant problem facing the financing of Chinese health care, even though there have been substantial improvements since 2000. Between 2000 and 2011, THE increased by 17.4% annually. During this same period, OOP payments as a percentage of THE declined from 53% to 38% (Long et al., 2013). This decrease in OOP expenditure is certainly welcome, but a persistent rural–urban divide remains. In urban areas, OOP payments as a percentage of total annual consumption was 6.4% in 2000; it rose to 7.6% by 2005 and fell again to 6.4% by 2011 (Long et al., 2013). In contrast, OOP payments rose from 5.2% to 8.4% of annual living expenses for rural areas, and surpassed urban areas in 2009. Even when comparing cities of varying wealth, urban residents still paid less, decreasing each year (Fig. 6.1) (Long et al., 2013). Among rural residents there is an upwards trend in the proportion of OOP health expenditure (Fig. 6.2) (Long et al., 2013). The gap may be driven by more generous urban insurance packages and a faster increase in urban incomes. The existence of this inequality and the fact that almost 10% of rural residents' spending is on OOP health care is concerning.

A significant proportion of Chinese households also face catastrophic health expenditures (Meng et al., 2012): this was 12.2%, 14.0% and 12.9% in 2003, 2008 and 2011, respectively. For rural households, the proportions were 13.6%, 15.1% and 13.8%, respectively.

Fig. 6.1 OOP health expenditure as a percentage of total income among urban residents by development level, 2005–2011

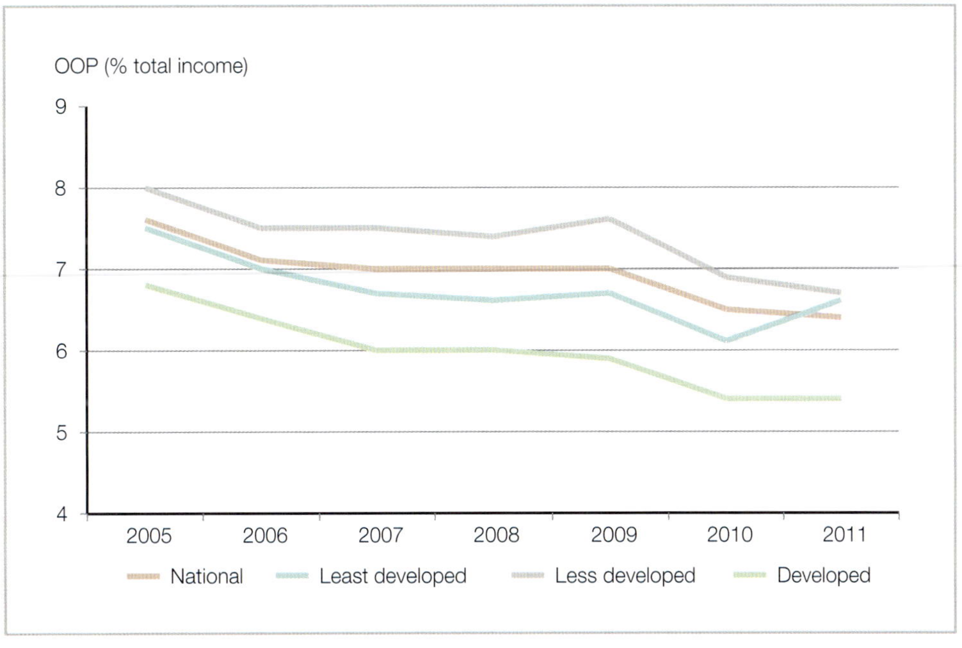

Source: Based on data in Long et al., 2013.

Fig. 6.2 OOP health expenditure as a percentage of total income among rural residents, 2005–2011

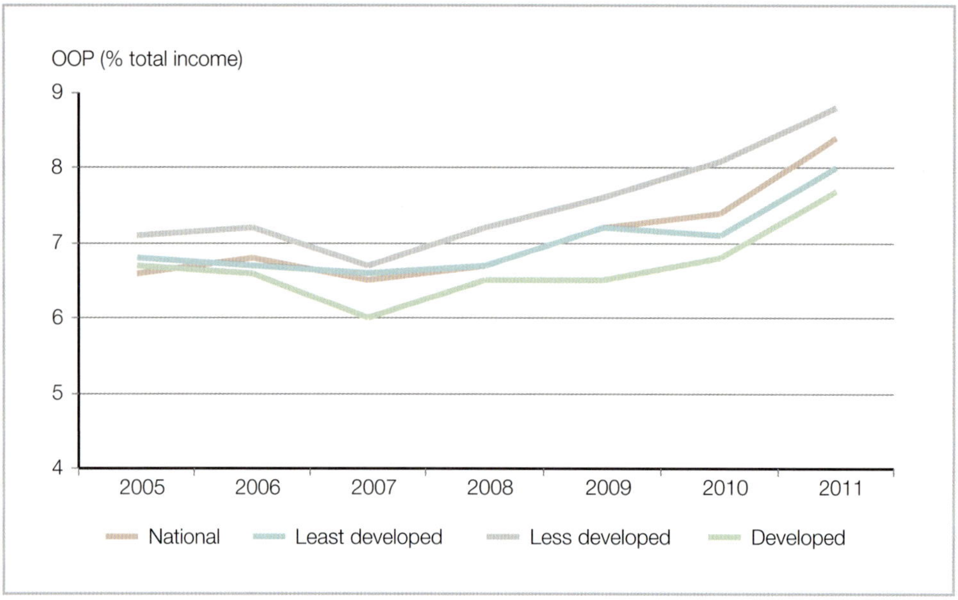

Source: Based on data in Long et al., 2013.

For urban households, the proportions were 9.0%, 11.3% and 10.9%, respectively. These numbers again highlight the higher burden faced by rural residents as well as the lack of any significant declines in catastrophic expenditures between 2003 and 2011.

There have also been studies on the price of a course of medication as a percentage of various daily reference standard wages. Different reference wages that have been used include the national poverty line in 2007 (RMB 1067/year), the per capita net income of a farmer and the wage of the lowest unskilled government worker (Jiang et al., 2013, 2014; Yang H et al., 2010).

Overall, medicines were found to be generally affordable, with most costing a day's wage or less for a standard course of treatment. In all cases, originator brands were more expensive than generics, in some cases costing as much as 14.5 days of wages for a standard treatment (e.g. for omeprazole, a gastrointestinal medication). Drugs for chronic conditions tended to be less affordable than those for acute conditions (Jiang et al., 2014). Affordability was also highly correlated with availability.

However, it is important to note that half of the medicines would require a day's income for the poorest people (those at the 2007 poverty line). Consequently, the financial burden may be high for a substantial portion of the population. Furthermore, some medicines were entirely unavailable as generic formulations or could not be found in the public sector at all. As originator brands and private sector medications tend to be much more expensive, affordability was quite low, with some medicines costing up to 11 days of wages for a course of treatment (e.g. atorvastatin, a cholesterol-lowering medication).

6.4 Availability of medications

The same studies that examined drug affordability in Hubei and Shaanxi also studied the availability of drugs at public and private outlets. The availability of essential drugs was generally fairly low. From the selection of medicines surveyed, in Hubei Province only 38.9% of the basket of drugs were available overall in public facilities in 2007 and 44.4% in private outlets (Table 6.2) (Jiang et al., 2013, 2014; Wang X et al., 2014b; Yang H et al., 2010). In Shaanxi Province, overall availability was also generally low for both adult and paediatric medications.

Private facilities have better drug availability than public ones for adult medications. This is unfortunate as the prices at private facilities tend to be higher than in public ones. Paediatric essential medications also demonstrate low availability. However, availability is higher for generics at public facilities than private ones for paediatric drugs. For all types of medication, availability for generics is much higher than for off-patent originators. Drugs for some important chronic conditions, such as metformin for diabetes and any

Table 6.2 Mean availability of generics and originator brands in public and private outlets

	2007 (Hubei, both generic and originator)	2010 (Shaanxi)	2012 (Shaanxi)	2012 (Shaanxi, paediatric drugs)
Generic drugs (% available)				
Public outlets	38.9	26.5	20.0	27.3
Private outlets	–	43.6	29.2	20.6
Off-patent originators (% available)				
Public outlets	44.4	8.9	7.1	10.8
Private outlets	–	18.1	12.6	11.9

Sources: Jiang et al., 2013, 2014; Wang X et al., 2014b; Yang H et al., 2010.

medications for mental health problems, were rare in both provinces. This suggests that patients with certain conditions would find it difficult to obtain the required medicines at all. Also worrisome is the fact that there was no increase in availability in Shaanxi Province between 2010 and 2012 even as the EDL should have been more broadly implemented.

In summary, there is generally poor availability of medicines, particularly in the public sector. While it is good that the private sector has higher availability so that more medicines are at least available somewhere, higher prices create access barriers. Additionally, many drugs for certain conditions have very low or no availability at all. Fortunately, generic drugs are more available than their much costlier off-patent originator counterparts. The low availability of EDL medications in 2012 is particularly concerning. Ultimately, these studies shed light on the fact that at least in the sample sites there are issues with accessibility even for relatively basic medications.

6.5 Conclusions

Addressing issues of medication affordability and accessibility is an important part of health care reform. Various studies have sought to assess the prices of medications compared with an international reference standard. While generic medications are reasonably priced, the off-patent originators are quite expensive. Finally, many medications are not available in generic formulation, at a public facility or simply at all. Hopefully, broader roll-out of the EDL will mean that the availability of basic medications increases. It is important that low-price generics are available in public facilities to help to improve affordability.

OOP health care expenditure remains quite high and is close to 10% of total spending for rural residents. While OOP expenditure is decreasing for urban residents, it is alarming that it is increasing for rural residents. Catastrophic health expenditure is also higher for rural households than urban ones. While many courses of drug treatment do cost less than a reference day's wages, some treatments can be many multiples of this standard. Improving affordability and access will be complex and will require concerted policy action and stronger government investment, particularly in rural areas. The introduction of novel pricing and reimbursement policies, the promotion of primary care, hospital reforms and the growing market for retail pharmacies will hopefully work synergistically to improve affordability and access. The most important move will be to increase the depth of health insurance coverage and perhaps even to harmonize the three different schemes.

7. Pharmaceutical pricing and reimbursement

KEY MESSAGES

- Pricing and reimbursement policies can be classified into supply-side policies, proxy-demand policies and demand-side policies. These policies have all had a number of expected effects but also unintended consequences.
- Pricing and reimbursement policies in China are currently undergoing significant changes, with different models set to replace the price ceilings that have largely been ineffective at cost-containment.
- Tendering is China's strongest and most effective pricing policy and has been successful at decreasing prices, especially for EDL drugs. However, concerns about quality have arisen and tendering more heavily weighted towards quality rather than just price is prudent until the overall level of pharmaceutical manufacturing improves.
- Reimbursement caps (a type of IRP) are set to replace retail price ceilings and have the potential to narrow the gap in price between off-patent originators and generic drugs. Little progress has been made with IRP or value-based pricing.
- As there is a lack of a national pharmaceutical framework, different provinces are experimenting with different pricing and reimbursement models. This is particularly apparent in the different tendering practises of individual provinces.
- Use of the EDL should be encouraged and its value as a percentage of all sales is set to increase dramatically over the next few years with expansion to higher-level health facilities.
- A six-year delay since the last NRDL update means that many newer medications are not currently insured.
- Local protectionism is a barrier to a more coherent pharmaceutical pricing and procurement strategy, as provinces will often favour local manufacturers when selecting who wins tenders. Increasing tender transparency and having more interprovince tenders can help to combat protectionism.

7.1 Context of pricing and reimbursement in China

Pricing and reimbursement is one of the most rapidly evolving aspects of pharmaceutical policy in China. It sits at the centre of what an effective and cohesive national pharmaceutical policy aims to do: provide quality medications at accessible prices while rewarding companies to promote the sustainable development of a strong local generic and R&D industry.

Prior to the 1978 market liberalization reforms, almost all drug prices were set by the government in China's centrally planned economy (World Bank, 2010). Market liberalization reforms led to a shift towards a private, market-oriented health care system. Government funding for health care declined precipitously. In order for hospitals and physicians to recoup lost revenue, they were allowed to charge a 15% mark-up on the sales of drugs, medical devices and diagnostic tests (Blumenthal & Hsiao, 2005).

This 15% mark-up created a cascade of negative consequences that policies are still aiming to rectify. It incentivized physicians and hospitals to offer more treatments, costlier treatments and inappropriate treatments. As basic physician salaries are low in China, physicians seek to supplement their income through drug sales, which are linked to bonuses and kickbacks (Development Research Center of the State Council, 2014). The phrase *yi yao yang yi* (drugs pay for doctors) is commonly heard in health care and aptly describes a system where 40% of THE is spent on pharmaceuticals but much of this money is actually going to pay doctors and hospital costs. Following the rapid privatization of China's health care system, drug prices grew at more than double digit rates annually. In response, the government set price ceilings on different products. Between 1997 and 2013, more than 30 price controls were announced (Wu, Zhang & Qiao, 2014) on a variety of drugs. Over the years, price ceilings were found to be largely ineffective and in the autumn of 2014 the NDRC announced that retail price ceilings would be eliminated from 1 June 2015.

7.2 How drugs go from market authorization to patients

It is helpful to have an understanding of how medications reach patients (Fig. 7.1). The first step is receiving approval and market authorization from the CFDA. After approval, drugs can be listed on one of the two major reimbursements lists: the EDL or the larger NRDL. Recently, China has begun to introduce major diseases schemes that cover more serious medical conditions and more expensive medications.

Drug pricing is largely determined through tendering for off-patent drugs or direct negotiations for patent drugs, with the NHFPC as a lead. The discussion on tendering will focus on hospitals as this is where most medications are purchased. After tender winners are announced, individual hospitals engage with individual manufacturers in a process known as secondary negotiation. During this process, actual drug volumes are specified and hospitals secure a price that is often lower than the listed tender price. Not all provinces engage in secondary negotiation. Finally, hospitals sell drugs directly to patients

Fig. 7.1 Drug movement from market authorization to patient use

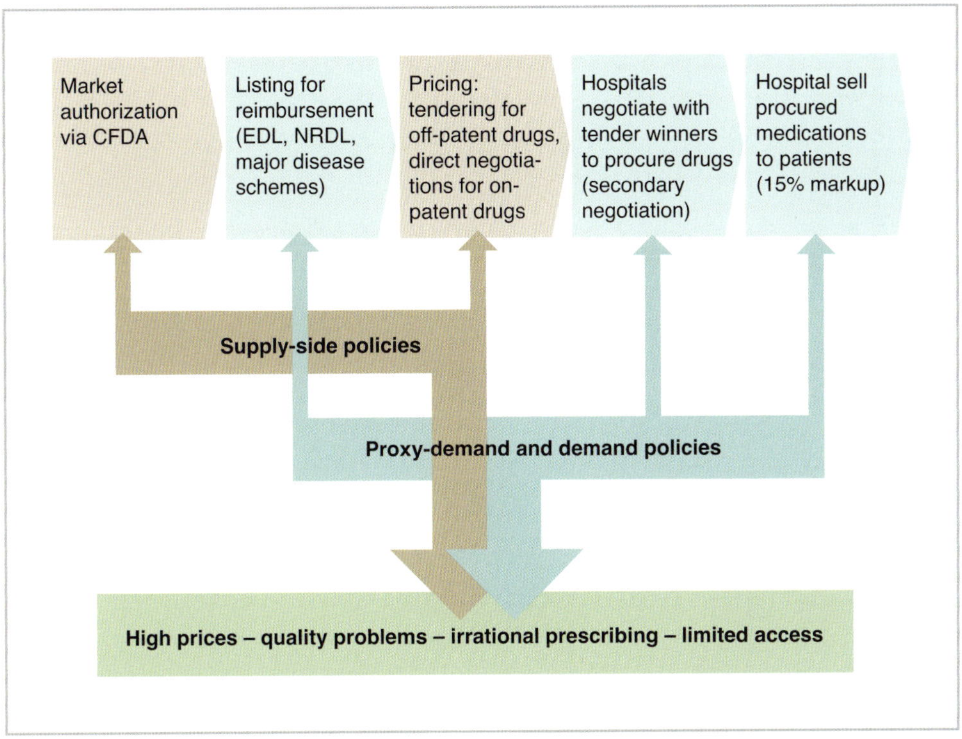

and can charge a 15% mark-up from what they had to pay. Multiple distributors exist between the manufacturers and hospital and these all charge mark-ups along the supply chain. The process is slightly different for primary care facilities and pharmacies. Provinces will directly procure for all its primary care facilities from tender winners while pharmacies are able to bypass the tender process and negotiate directly with manufacturers (Development Research Center of the State Council, 2015).

Pricing and reimbursement policies in China can be classified in terms of supply-side policies as well as proxy-demand polices and demand-side policies. Supply-side policies include both the market authorization process and drug quality regulations as well as direct pricing policies such as price controls and tendering. Proxy-demand policies refer to factors that influence health care providers (who act as proxies for patients in deciding what drugs to use), such as the 15% mark-up. Demand-side policies refer to factors that directly influence patient demand, such as reimbursement lists. This section will focus specifically on direct pricing and reimbursement policies, leaving the effects of market authorization and drug quality policies to be covered in other chapters. An overview of these policies, along with their intended and unintended consequences is presented in Table 7.1.

Table 7.1 Summary of supply-side, proxy-demand and demand-side policies

Policy environment	Policy initiatives	Expected effects	Unintended consequences
Supply-side policies			
Drug application backlog	Caused by fragmented manufacturing system driving too many applications; CFDA recently promised to resolve backlog	Significant delays in approval of all drugs	Delays in approving drugs that are clinically superior or needed generics lead to health and economic costs
Low drug quality	Successively more stringent standards for GMP and bioequivalence testing have been introduced	Presence of large number of low-quality domestic generics on the market that are not equivalent to off-patent originators and can be harmful to patients	Creation of significant price difference between off-patent originator drugs and domestic generics
Price ceilings	Used extensively in the past, eliminated in 2015	Intended to contain drug prices	Easy to evade by registering new drugs or higher-volume prescribing
Tendering	Primary mechanism by which off-patent drugs are priced	Price reductions following the introduction of tendering	Excessive reliance on price leads to a "race-to-the-bottom" with significant quality concerns

Table 7.1 Summary of supply-side, proxy-demand and demand-side policies (continued)

Policy environment	Policy initiatives	Expected effects	Unintended consequences
HTA/CER	Exploratory analysis has been carried out but policy use is limited	Could theoretically promote rational prescribing and prioritize which drugs need approval	
International reference pricing	Exploratory analysis has been carried out but not formalized into policy	Could theoretically help benchmark Chinese prices to international ones and lead to price reductions	
Negotiations for patent drugs	Primary mechanism by which patent drugs are priced; NHFPC is currently formulating national guidelines	Formulating national guidelines could increase transparency of negotiations	
Proxy-demand policies			
Secondary negotiation	Required for hospitals to procure drugs from manufacturers; current debate around where difference between tender price and secondary negotiation price should accrue	Allows hospitals to specify volumes of drug procured and often leads to prices lower than the listed tender prices	If earnings accrue to hospitals, this may incentivize drug-related revenues
15% mark-up	Found throughout health care system, although recent efforts have been made to remove the mark-up	Intended to help hospitals and physicians to have another source of income following decreases in government funding	Prescribing of expensive drugs and unnecessary drugs

Table 7.1 Summary of supply-side, proxy-demand and demand-side policies (continued)

Policy environment	Policy initiatives	Expected effects	Unintended consequences
Low hospital funding and physicians salaries	Hospitals receive little direct government funding and physicians are paid quite poorly	Hospitals and physicians will look for revenue from other avenues	Reliance on drug sales for revenue fosters environment where bribery and kickbacks from industry can flourish
ZMU	Introduced in 2009 reforms and implemented in primary care facilities and half of county hospitals; to be implemented at all city hospitals in 2017	Removes perverse incentive to over-prescribe associated with the 15% mark-up	Without sufficient government subsidies, increased provision of medical services for revenue encouraged
Demand-side policies			
EDL	Introduced in 2009 reforms along with ZMU; intended for broadened rollout	Ensures that a basic set of drugs is available and accessible	Lack of HTA/CER does not encourage rational drug choice
NRDL	Introduced in 2000, last updated in 2009; broader reimbursement with class A (more important) and class B (less important) medications	Primary drug reimbursement list in China	Gaps in coverage and delays in update lead to problems with access and affordability; lack of HTA/CER does not encourage rational drug choice
Reimbursement caps	Introduced in 2015 to replace price ceilings to promote rational prescribing; not yet implemented	Could theoretically promote rational prescribing and drug quality through financial incentives	

7.3 Supply-side policies

7.3.1 Price ceilings and price cuts

China has used price ceilings and cuts set by the NDRC for many years. There is a substantial body of evidence that suggests that these have been ineffective in containing drug costs. While the prices of targeted drugs have decreased by an average of 15–20% and as much as 60%, TPE has still steadily increased (Wu, Zhang & Qiao, 2014). One study looked at the effect of four price caps on antibiotic costs in 12 Beijing hospitals between 1996 and 2005 (Han et al., 2013). While the prices of targeted antibiotics were 47% less in 2005 than 1996, overall expenditure on antibiotics was 205.7% higher in 2005. The authors suggested that physicians can easily evade price ceilings by switching to more expensive antibiotics or prescribing higher doses of medication. Similar results are reported in another study that used macroeconomic data to look at the effects of price regulations (Wu, Zhang & Qiao, 2014). The authors found that, while there was a slight initial decrease in pharmaceutical price indexes, the regulations did not reduce household expenditure on drugs or the profitability of pharmaceutical firms. Price regulations also cause an increase in the importation of more expensive foreign-produced medication. Essentially, physicians incentivized by the 15% mark-up have largely been able to evade the effects of direct price regulations.

The ability of providers to offer more expensive alternatives was made easier by the fact that price ceilings often only affected specific formulations or brand names of a medication, meaning it would be easy to switch to another company's product or formulation. Manufacturers could even evade price regulations by registering a "new drug" that was really the same old drug with very minor alterations or even just a changed name (World Bank, 2010). New CFDA regulations aim to prevent registrations of such phony "new drugs".

During the era of price regulation, studies showed that competition could effectively lower prices. A study of hospital drug costs across China between 1999 and 2002 found that local generic competition served to drive down the prices of generics but not of imported medications (Wang, 2006). The perception of non-substitutability between imported and generic drugs is a reflection of quality concerns. Another study looking at 11 tertiary hospitals between 2002 and 2005 found that the prices of medications were negatively correlated with the number of generic alternatives but positively correlated with the number of therapeutic classes to treat a condition (Wu J et al., 2014). The former suggests that competition does drive down prices. The latter finding comes from the fact that drugs from different therapeutic classes can obtain patent protection and thus command price premiums.

The era of formal price ceilings came to an end on June 1, 2015. However, mandated price cuts in subsequent rounds of tendering appear to be continuing in many provinces. In conjunction with price ceiling elimination, there will be a six-month period of enhanced surveillance of drug market pricing activities. During this period, the government has planned ad hoc inspections of drug pricing behaviour of all players in the pharmaceutical market along with a hotline that consumers can call regarding price complaints. Companies found to be engaged in "price-fixing" behaviour face the possibility of a two-year ban from the public procurement system (NDRC, 2014a).

Monitoring of drug prices following the removal of price ceilings is prudent given the significance of the policy change. While significant evidence suggests that price ceilings are not effective at long-term containment of overall drug expenditure, they have been able to yield short-term savings (Carone, Schwierz & Xavier, 2012; Mossialos, Mrazek & Walley, 2004). Therefore, it is theoretically possible that removal of direct price controls can result in short-term price increases. For example, the consumer hotline yielded 442 complaints regarding drug pricing in the month of June (11ey.com, 2015). Another media report suggested that a majority of off-patent obstetric/gynaecological and paediatric medications increased in price, with increases in the range of 100% to 200% from the last tender round (Sai, 2015b). In general, all the polices being introduced and experimented with should be closely monitored and evaluated in order to guide future decision-making.

7.3.2 Tendering

Tendering is now the main strategy used by governments to price drugs. After the removal of direct price controls, tendering is effectively the only cost-containment strategy available for off-patent drugs. While reimbursement caps are being implemented, tendering will definitely be China's most important pricing policy.

Tendering is the primary mechanism by which provinces acquire medications for the EDL and is also used for many NRDL drugs. Companies must win tenders to sell that drug within a province and the government mandates that health care institutions must purchase a majority of their medications (around 80% by value) from winning tender lists (Yang & Lei, 2010). Therefore, winning tenders is crucial for the survival of drug manufacturers. Tendering has been successful at lowering EDL drug prices by 25% on average and over 50% in some provinces between 2009 and 2010 (Hu, 2013). It is also generally accepted that each subsequent round of tendering will lead to a decline in the price of a medication, with mandated price cuts from the previous tender winner levels (Development Research Center of the State Council, 2015).

Tendering is carried out separately by each of China's provinces, many of which use different tendering criteria. Since 2010, variations on Anhui Province's "two-envelope" system have been broadly employed: the first envelope is one of quality (defined in many different ways) and the second envelope is that of price (lowest price wins). Traditionally, the Anhui model has been heavily weighted towards price, but these weights can vary significantly by province (Development Research Center of the State Council, 2015). Furthermore, in some provinces, only one company can win a tender for a particular drug while in others there can be up to three winners (Development Research Center of the State Council, 2015). There is also significant variation in the different tiers of tendered drugs. Most provinces tender off-patent originators separately from generic medications, with the assumption that the originators are of higher quality, while a few will put these in the same tender. For example, Hubei and Sichuan uses four categories for EDL tendering while Guangdong only has one category, making no distinctions in quality (McTiernan, 2014a). In general, off-patent originators are able to command a large price premium over locally produced generics. A study demonstrated average price differences of 40%, but anecdotally off-patent originators can be as much as ten times the cost of generics (Hu et al., 2015; Jiang et al., 2013, 2014).

In spite of its ability to lower prices, tendering has received many criticisms. One of the main criticisms has been an excessive emphasis on price over quality, leading to major problems with quality (Development Research Center of the State Council, 2015). What this means is that manufacturers of low-quality products are able to undercut those producing high-quality drugs on the basis of price, leading to a race to the bottom in terms of drug quality. Another criticism has been the fact that tenders tend to be awarded entirely to one company. This leads to monopolies and shortages if the company runs into any production difficulties (Barber et al., 2013). Tenders are also not linked with procurement so hospitals must negotiate specific volumes and prices with manufacturers via secondary negotiation after the tendering process (Development Research Center of the State Council, 2015). Based on these criticisms, China's tendering system is currently undergoing significant changes. In the first half of 2015, both the State Council and the NHFPC released several key policy guidance documents regarding the tendering process (NHFPC, 2015; State Council, 2015b).

Proper quality assessment is one of the most important aspects of tendering reform (Development Research Center of the State Council, 2015). In developed countries with more advanced pharmaceutical markets, generics are considered to be of identical quality to originators based on strict bioequivalence testing and GMP standards. Improving generic quality would go a long way in narrowing the price premium commanded by off-patent originators. Unfortunately, because of shortcomings with bioequivalence testing and GMP standards in China, actual quality assessment is difficult. For example, Beijing's quality assessment scorecard is composed of 15 evaluation items, most of which are based on company reputation, revenues and industrial ranking as determined by the government ministries rather than objective quality data (Table 7.2) (McTiernan, 2014a).

In spite of the trend towards more quality-oriented tendering, in the most recent round of 2015 tendering in Hunan and Zhejiang Provinces there was significant acrimony from drug manufacturers because of aggressive government mandated price cuts (McTiernan, 2015d). In Hunan, EDL and non-EDL drugs were tendered together through direct online price competition or price negotiations. The negotiations apparently involved pricing experts establishing a price that companies could accept or refuse, with the latter being understood as a withdrawal from the tender. Meanwhile, in Zhejiang Province there was an across-the-board 10% price cut followed by further cuts for specific products and the top-selling 200 drugs. It appears likely that other provinces will emulate the aggressive price cuts demanded by these provinces as their tender contracts come up.

Table 7.2 Beijing tendering quality scorecard

	Evaluation criteria	Weighting
Manufacturer size	Quality assurance (GMP)	3
	Company ranking by MIIT	10
	Annual turnover	15
	Innovation (as recognized in China)	12
	Local investment	5
	Corporate brand (from knowledge leaders)	5
Product quality	Quality specification	5
	Differential pricing category from NDRC	10
	Product line/formulation quality (GMP)	5
	Tender winning record	10
	Active Pharmaceutical Ingredient quality control (GMP)	2
	Output ranking by MIIT	10
	Electronic monitoring	3
	Product reputation (from knowledge leaders)	5
Additional	Negative quality reports	-10

Source: McTiernan, 2014a.

Note: MIIT: Ministry of Industry and Information Technology.

With tendering processes evolving so quickly and with so much provincial variation, it remains to be seen what the most effective policies will be and if a dominant mechanism will evolve that will be promoted nationally. The move towards web-based tendering in multiple provinces may pave the way for a national tendering and procurement strategy. Already, many new tenders call for price ceilings based on average or lowest tender prices in previous tenders across the country (Development Research Center of the State Council, 2015). One effect of this provincial reference pricing is that drug companies are keen to keep prices the same across provinces in order to avoid price cuts. This does not make sense from a health care or economic perspective given the vastly different buying power of the provinces. An advantage of a more nationally coordinated tendering strategy would be a tiered-pricing structure in which the poorer provinces pay less and the wealthier provinces more.

Another important part of centralized electronic tendering is that it would help to combat local protectionism. When provinces use tenders individually, it is easy for authorities to favour local manufacturers. However, this would be more difficult if tendering was carried out by groups of provinces or by the country as a whole. Finally, electronic tendering, which minimizes face-to-face interaction, can mitigate against bribery and other types of influence that have helped to drive local protectionism.

There has also been an emphasis on greater transparency, not only of winning tender prices but also of secondary negotiation prices, which have in the past been confidential (Pharmnet, 2015). Shanghai, Beijing and Zhejiang were some of the first jurisdictions to introduce more transparent procurement (Sai, 2015c). As these prices are the ones hospitals actually pay, they are essential to having useful price comparisons (Development Research Center of the State Council, 2015).

7.3.3 International reference pricing and negotiations for patent drugs

In 2012, the NDRC asked a number of multinational drug companies to provide prices for their products in 10 international markets. This survey revealed that, while 60% of drugs fell within the international price range, half were in the upper half of drug prices (Development Research Center of the State Council, 2014). Furthermore, 20% of drugs were more expensive in China than anywhere else in the world. In July 2015, the NDRC released a document suggesting that multinational corporations will soon have to provide drug prices in the home country as well as prices in the United Kingdom, France, the Netherlands, 12 other European countries, the United States and markets in Asia and Africa (NDRC, 2015). There has been no formal announcement of international reference pricing, but collection of these data could pave the way for such a system. These prices could potentially inform maximum allowable prices for provincial tenders

While the patented drugs market is small, at less than 10% of total market value, the market is projected to grow rapidly, particularly as major disease schemes are implemented and insurance coverage levels increase (Boston Consulting Group, 2014). For patented drugs, the NHFPC is formulating national guidelines for price negotiations. Historical procurement and retail prices will be combined with international and interprovince reference prices to create reference points for price negotiations (McTiernan, 2015d). There are also plans for formalization of price–volume agreements, which have often been lacking in China.

7.3.4 HTA and CER

HTA and CER are relatively new in China. The 2009 health care reforms called for greater use of health economic data when drug companies submit NDAs, but progress has been limited (Oortwijn, Mathijssen & Banta, 2010). In 2010, a memorandum of understanding was signed between the China National Health Development Research Center, the research arm of the NHFPC, and the United Kingdom National Institute of Health and Care Excellence, although much of the work has focused on clinical pathways and guidelines (Zhao, 2014). So far, HTA has been used in the assessment of major medical devices such as surgical robots and interventional procedures such as dialysis and organ transplantation (Meng et al., 2015).

The NHFPC is currently developing national HTA guidelines that could be institutionalized broadly (Meng et al., 2015). Provincially, Zhejiang's Health and Family Planning Commission has recently created a pharmacoeconomic evaluation committee to contribute to the pricing process for tenders (McTiernan, 2014a). In general, while HTA has been researched and piloted it is yet to be incorporated broadly into policy (Kennedy-Martin et al., 2014). CER looks at differences in clinical effectiveness between therapies without economic consideration. While it is less methodologically challenging than HTA, CER is also not used extensively in pricing or reimbursement decisions. HTA and CER could be incorporated into the drug pricing or reimbursement process to promote the use of effective and cost-efficient therapies.

7.4 Proxy-demand policies

7.4.1 Secondary negotiation

Secondary negotiation is necessary for quantifying volumes of drugs sold from manufacturers to hospitals, a process that also results in a price lower than listed tender winning prices. It is used in some provinces but not in others. The key issue surrounding secondary negotiations is where the cost difference between tender price and the secondary price will accrue: to hospitals and physicians or a central government agency. Empowering hospitals to negotiate aggressively and to keep the cost savings is seen as promoting efficiency in negotiations. However, there is a concern that this will be yet another incentive to purchase and then prescribe more expensive drugs in order to capture greater savings, in a manner not dissimilar to the 15% mark-up (Development Research Center of the State Council, 2015). Because of this, secondary negotiation has been controversial. The NDRC and the Ministry of Human Resources and Social Security have been supportive and launched various pilots where such negotiations are carried out openly, while the

NHFPC has generally been opposed (Development Research Center of the State Council, 2015). This concern led the NHFPC to issue Document 70 in June 2015, calling for either a ban on secondary negotiations or at least for the savings to accrue to governments (NHPFC, 2015). The issue of secondary negotiations is still being contested in China.

7.4.2 The 15% mark-up and ZMU policies

The 15% mark-up policy has been the key proxy-demand factor that encourages over-prescribing. The ZMU policy, a ban on the mark-up health care facilities are allowed to charge on medications, was introduced in 2009 to combat the perverse incentives created by the 15% mark-up. It was intended to remove the link between drug prescribing and health care facility income.

ZMU has almost universally been implemented in primary care facilities. Currently, over half of county hospitals and dozens of urban hospitals have also implemented ZMU (Ellis, 2015). In the 2015 health care reform work plan, the State Council called for all county hospitals and all urban hospitals to implement ZMU by 2015 and 2017, respectively (State Council, 2015d). Since so much hospital revenue comes from drug sales, implementation will be extremely challenging. It will require significant increases in either direct government subsidies or revenue generated from the provision of medical services.

At the primary care level, ZMU has led to significant declines in drug revenues for health providers (Table 7.3). However, government subsidies have not been sufficient to make-up for the lost drug revenues, which puts into question the long-term sustainability of ZMU (Hu, 2013; Zhang X et al., 2014). There have also been some improvements in affordability and decreased irrational prescribing (Chen et al., 2014; Song et al., 2014b; Xiang et al., 2012). Interestingly, there is also evidence that inpatient visits have increased in order to make-up for lost revenue (Yi et al., 2015). County-level hospitals implementing ZMU have also seen declines in drug revenues. As with primary care facilities, government subsidies and medical service fee rates have not made up for these losses (Zhou Z et al., 2015a). Furthermore, there were increases in the provision of both inpatient and outpatient services (Zhou Z et al., 2015b). There have been few evaluations of ZMU in urban hospitals although a recent announcement by the NHFPC, the Ministry of Finance and the State Council on an evaluation of urban hospital pilots hinted at mixed results in reducing overprescribing incentive and lowering patient costs (Wang, 2015).

Table 7.3 Summary of effects of ZMU policies by level of health care facility

Level of health care facility	Effects
Primary care[a]	Multiple studies demonstrate decreases in drug revenues; some evidence of decreases in drug prices and in irrational prescribing; some evidence of increased service provision
County-level hospitals[b]	Decrease in drug revenue with increases in service-related revenue and government subsidies that do not fully compensate; some evidence of increased service provision
Higher-tier hospitals[c]	Unclear; latest reports on pilot projects suggest mixed results

Sources:
[a] Xiang et al., 2012; Hu, 2013; Chen et al., 2014; Song et al., 2014b; Zhang X et al., 2014; Yi et al., 2015;
[b] Zhou Z et al., 2015a, 2015b;
[c] Wang, 2015.

7.5 Demand-side policies

7.5.1 EDL

The creation of an essential medications list was one of the five pillars of the health care reforms. The list was designed to guarantee a supply of safe quality drugs at affordable prices and to deter irrational prescribing. It was initially meant for primary care facilities, with the eventual goal of expansion to hospitals (Yip et al., 2012). The EDL was first created in 2009 and updated in 2012. China has experimented with essential medication lists in the past (Guan et al., 2011). The first such list was actually created in 1982 and was updated five times prior to 2009, with the 2004 update containing 2001 items. Prior to 2009, these essential medication lists lacked policy support in drug production, distribution, pricing and reimbursement and were not integrated into the broader health system. The new EDL was meant to take these factors into consideration and to be a tool for health care reform. Criteria for listing include clinical necessity, efficacy, safety and affordability. The EDL is also a generics drug list, meaning that off-patent originators could have much higher price ceilings than the EDL molecule (Guan et al., 2011).

The 2009 EDL contained 205 western and 102 TCM drugs. However, provinces were allowed to supplement this initial list considerably: 3 provinces added more than 200 items, 16 added 100–200, 10 added 0–100, and 2 added none. A study using the

DELPHI method with five pharmacy experts and five senior general practitioners found that medications on the core EDL were generally appropriately selected based on listing criteria but those on the supplemental lists often were not (Tian, Song & Zhang, 2012). The revised EDL saw an expansion to 317 western and 203 TCM medications, with the government stipulating that there should be less provincial adjustment.

Through tendering, the EDL appears to have been successful at decreasing drug prices (Hu, 2013; Tian, Song & Zhang, 2012). An evaluation of the EDL in three provinces in China found that prices had decreased and that there was less irrational prescribing, but that reliability of drug supplies and the income of primary care facilities had fallen (Li Y et al., 2013). In terms of availability, a few studies in the centrally located Shaanxi Province demonstrated relatively low availability (uniformly <50%) of a sample of EDL medications in both 2010 and 2012 (Jiang et al., 2013, 2014).

In principle, EDL medications are fully covered (with no deductibles) by all three of China's insurance schemes. In practice, what is actually covered depends on the local jurisdiction and is often a city- or county-level decision. The UEBMI tends to be the most generous and well funded and the NCMS the least generous and least well funded. There are also distinctions made between inpatient and outpatient coverage for EDL, with the former generally being better reimbursed than the latter. Extensive regional variations exist: the wealthiest areas such as Shanghai and Beijing have much lower deductibles and higher reimbursement ceilings than poorer cities. In the latest 2015 State Council work plan, a target of at least 50% coverage for outpatient and 75% coverage for inpatient care across all three insurance schemes has been set (State Council, 2015d). The government sees the EDL playing an increasing role in China's pharmaceutical system. By the end of 2020, it is estimated that the EDL will make up 28% of China's drug market by value, an increase from 12% in 2011 (Boston Consulting Group, 2014).

7.5.2 NRDL

The NRDL is an older, larger and less standardized list than the EDL. It differs from the EDL in that reimbursement rates are generally lower, there is not yet mandatory implementation of ZMU for NRDL drugs and different ministries manage the lists (EDL is managed by the NHFPC while NRDL is managed by the Ministry of Human Resources and Social Security). The first iteration of the NRDL was created in 2000, with updates in 2004 and 2009. The 2009 version contains 1140 western and 987 TCM medications and is divided into two classes (Yoongthong et al., 2012). Class A (349 western, 154 TCM) drugs are seen as effective, essential and relatively cheap and are supposed to be fully reimbursable. Class B (791 western, 833 TCM) drugs are considered less essential and have different co-payments depending on the province. These reimbursement amounts generally apply to the urban insurance schemes, with the UEBMI again being more generous than the URBMI. Provinces create their own lists based on the NRDL. All class A drugs must be on provincial lists but 15% of class B medications can be adjusted to suit local needs. Provinces also formulate a list of drugs covered under NCMS, which tends to be far less extensive than what is covered under the urban plans. The differences in provincial NRDL lists and differences between the urban and NCMS schemes mean that the degree of actual drug coverage varies significantly across the country.

The NRDL was meant to be updated every two years, with thousands of national and provincial experts participating in a complex voting process (Ngorsuraches et al., 2012). For the most recent 2009 update, the Ministry of Human Resources and Social Security chaired the final selection group, which contained representatives from the NDRC, the State Food and Drug Administration (the old version of the CFDA), the State Administration of Traditional Chinese Medicine, Ministry of Civil Affairs, Ministry of Finance and Ministry of Industry and Information Technology. The lengthy time between NRDL updates means that new drugs experience significant delays between approval and reimbursement (IMS Health, 2014b). Due to the lack of updates since 2009, no new medications approved since then have been added to the NRDL. As a result, of 360 new drugs approved in China between 2003 and 2013, only 76 (21%) are on the NRDL (IMS Health, 2014b). Medications not on the NRDL or EDL must be paid for as OOP payment.

7.5.3 Major disease schemes

Major disease schemes are emerging as a way to cover costly medical conditions. They provide supplementary coverage on top of basic medical insurance reimbursement limits for conditions that have novel and costly medicines, such as cancer and autoimmune disorders. The government is considering having these schemes operated by private insurance companies (Meng et al., 2015). In July 2015, Premier Li Keqiang announced at a State Council Summit that provincial pilots for major disease schemes should be expanded nationally by the end of 2015, with minimum 50% coverage, and that there should be full implementation by the end of 2017 (Xue, 2015).

7.5.4 Reimbursement caps

Reimbursement caps are a form of IRP that are intended to replace the now defunct price ceilings. Under the new system, responsibility for drug pricing, formerly primarily the responsibility of the NDRC, would be shared by the Ministry of Human Resources and Social Security and the NHFPC (McTiernan, 2015d). As a result, the influence of the NDRC has weakened compared with the other ministries involved in health care.

Previously, in 2011, the NDRC created a draft proposal for IRP for NRDL medications. Under the initial plan, there would still be different classes of drug based on perceived quality (e.g. patented drugs, off-patent originators, first-to-market generics). Sanming City in Fujian Province, one of the country's leading health care reformers, adopted a more aggressive policy. Reimbursement caps were placed on 14 molecules felt to have only minor quality differences between domestic generic and imported versions but that exhibited large price gaps. Caps were set at the price of the cheapest domestically manufactured generic – much lower than off-patent originator prices. This move led to significant voluntary price reductions from multinational corporations (McTiernan, 2015d).

However, it seems unlikely that a policy that does not take into account quality would be broadly adopted given the current emphasis being placed on improving drug quality.

Although the government is encouraging the use of reimbursement caps, actual implementation remains unclear. The delineation of responsibilities across ministries is one area of uncertainty. It does appear that the Ministry of Human Resources and Social Security will take the lead as it is the main payer through its management of the UEBMI and URBMI, although the NHFPC may also play an important role because of its purported expertise in health care (Development Research Center of the State Council, 2015). Another area of difficulty is how reimbursement levels will be set. A recent document from the NDRC's Academy of Macroeconomic Research suggests that drug costs, drug quality and winning tender prices could all be incorporated into reimbursement levels, but provides no clear guidance on what will actually be done (Academy of Macroeconomic Research, 2015).

7.6 Conclusions

There have been a number of developments in pricing and reimbursement in China over recent years. In general, there has been an orientation towards fewer direct price controls and more market-oriented strategies. China has been borrowing strategies from various international countries, particularly Germany, in setting up novel policies.

The most significant development has been the removal of the price ceilings that have been the norm for many years. These will be replaced with reimbursement caps that seek to minimize the gap between off-patent originators and generics, a move that will hopefully strengthen China's domestic generics industry. Tendering is also changing in a number of ways. There is a movement away from the largely price-driven tendering system to one that incorporates quality into winning bids. The use of online platforms will lead to greater transparency and the possibility of more interprovince linking for reference pricing and the possibility eventually of a national tendering system. For on-patent medications, new guidance should soon be released by the central government outlining how negotiations have transpired, but it is likely there will be movement towards price–volume agreements that engender price reductions for volume guarantees. IRP and HTA/CER have yet to be formally promulgated in any serious way, but it seems likely that these two areas will develop further over the next few years as China's drug market matures.

In terms of reimbursement, there will be a continued move to expand the EDL beyond primary care facilities and county hospitals, and market share is sure to increase. The next update of the EDL is soon due, and it will be interesting to see what new additions will be made, particularly with more expensive and potentially on-patent medications. Meanwhile, the NRDL has not yet been updated since 2009, meaning newer medications that are not on the EDL simply are not being reimbursed. This has created a drug reimbursement lag that, in combination with the regulatory delays from a backlogged CFDA, means many new medications are not reaching the population.

Creating a pricing and reimbursement system that is capable of encouraging cost-containment and quality of generics while simultaneously allowing for innovative new products to be reimbursed is a significant challenge. Removing ineffective price ceilings and using more market-oriented approaches and encouraging more EDL drug use are good first steps. Moving forwards, it will be essential for China to coordinate broader health care reforms with its drug pricing and reimbursement strategies and to engage in a more coherent national pharmaceutical policy formulation.

8. Drug quality and supply chain

KEY MESSAGES

- The CFDA needs significant strengthening of its capacity to carry out effective oversight of its drug approval and quality monitoring roles.
- Ensuring pharmaceutical quality is a pressing issue, as GMP guidelines are not aligned with international standards nor sufficiently enforced among manufacturers. This has led to both domestic and international scepticism of Chinese pharmaceutical quality.
- Bioequivalence testing has been weak in China, leading to vast differences in quality between generics and off-patent originators. The CFDA has recently introduced more stringent requirements to address this issue.
- Fragmentation among pharmaceutical producers exacerbates quality concerns. Reducing the number of major manufacturers will help to increase the size of existing firms, which should improve quality. Unfortunately, local protectionism has made consolidation of the pharmaceutical industry difficult.
- Again, fragmentation in the distribution chain means there are many mark-ups between production and patient use and access to medicines can be highly geographically dependent. Consolidation efforts through acquisition of smaller companies by larger national companies are underway.
- Addressing issues of quality control and decreasing fragmentation in the manufacturing and distribution chains will improve access to, and increase trust in, Chinese pharmaceuticals among Chinese and international consumers.

8.1 The role of the CFDA in drug quality

Historically, drug oversight has been by government agencies that have had a changing relationship with central government. These various regulatory bodies have faced a number of challenges in the past. For example, in 1998, the State Food and Drug Administration became separated from the Ministry of Health and reported directly to the State Council. Following concerns over lack of oversight, it was brought back under Ministry of Health control in 2008. Trust in the agency has also been affected by high-profile incidents concerning food and drug safety, as well as the execution of its former head for corruption (Yu et al., 2010). The current CFDA represents another attempt to make the drug regulatory agency independent, and it now again reports directly to the State Council (Qi, 2012). The most recent iteration of the CFDA has a comprehensive set of responsibilities including drug approval, standards and inspection, which hopefully means moving forwards it will be better able to guarantee the safety and quality of China's medications (Qi, 2012). While the CFDA has sole national oversight, its work is aided by provincial food and drug administrations.

As the pharmaceutical industry in China has expanded, there have been concerns about the agency's ability to cope with the regulatory workload. The volume of approved drugs has expanded significantly, from around 10 000 approved in 2004 to around 170 000 in 2008 (Qi, 2012). Concerns have been raised about the quality of the approval process, with some drugs gaining approval after only a name change or slight formulation changes (Qi, 2012; World Bank, 2010). Similarly, in the past, companies sought approval for new medications frequently to evade price cap regulation (World Bank, 2010). For all approved drugs, the CFDA also has the huge responsibility of ensuring drug quality. Re-elevating the CFDA to a full ministerial agency should give it more power to enforce quality regulation, and increased legal penalties for quality breaches should encourage compliance with existing legislation (Qi, 2012). An effective and independent drug regulation agency is essential in ensuring institutional responsiveness if it can overcome past issues of trust in the drug approval and quality process.

8.2 Quality standards in China

8.2.1 GMP

The proliferation of pharmaceutical manufacturers has led to diversification of manufacturing processes. In part because of an increasingly competitive market, manufacturers were rushed to spend their capital in the form of factories, in some cases with not enough money left over for oversight practices (Qi, 2012). These conditions make quality control difficult for manufacturers to prioritize. Limited CFDA capacity to conduct inspections further compounds the problem.

Manufacturers of finished drugs all require a GMP licence. However, some companies manufacture intermediate chemicals and Active Pharmaceutical Ingredients (APIs) and so do not require a GMP licence (and are not regulated in the same way) (Sun, 2007). Unfortunately, despite being widely required, there is considerable variation in how GMP is actually applied. Inspections show a number of areas of potential deficiency, such as process validation, documentation and quality assurance processes (Sun, 2007; Vincent, 2014). Additionally, there is little oversight of manufacturers of APIs more upstream in the manufacturing chain, which do not require a GMP licence. The variation in GMP produces strain at all levels of the manufacturing chain, as downstream manufacturers are faced with pressure to use lowest cost intermediary vendors, potentially sacrificing GMP standards. Chinese pharmaceutical firms have been oriented towards a domestic market, where GMP requirements are not as clear or as strict. This differs from foreign-oriented markets such as that in India, which has much better alignment with international GMP standards (Vincent, 2014). This results in varying quality of drug production a potential safety concern that worries both Chinese citizens and export markets.

A key concern in the adherence to GMP is the limited oversight and regulation capacity of the CFDA and its provincial affiliates. The CFDA has very few members of staff given the size of its regulatory responsibility. This has been addressed somewhat by increasing the clarity of GMP regulations, revising drug registration processes and increasing inspection (Sun, 2007). Legal controls for exported products have been strengthened by specific regulations that authorize the seizure of profits and products in the case of production of fakes, or neglecting product examination (Sun, 2007). This is a good start, but institutional inspection capacity should also be increased to ensure compliance at all stages of the manufacturing chain. In any given year, only a fraction of factories are actually inspected by the CFDA and its provincial counterparts. In 2014, the CFDA announced measures that would allow for unannounced site inspections of manufacturers and distributors (Covington and Burling LLP, 2014a). These measures would give both the CFDA and its provincial counterparts significantly broader discretion to perform inspections; if this was linked with enforcement, it would improve oversight. Hopefully CFDA's recent announcement of an increase in application fees for NDAs can also lead to more resources for its operation.

8.2.2 Drug quality and bioequivalence testing

Quality is an important issue in how Chinese patients choose to purchase their drugs. Most patients prefer to purchase their drugs from hospitals. There is the perception of higher quality, convenience and physician recommendation that influences this decision (Yu et al., 2010). Consumers tend to be influenced by perceptions of quality and proxy measures thereof, such as drug or store brand (Zhou, Xue & Ping, 2013).

The 2007 version of the Drug Registration Regulations included specifications for the treatment of generic drugs, where a generic is defined as a drug previously approved by the CFDA (Rizzi & Lin, 2011). Similar to developed countries, generics are subject to less stringent testing compared with new drugs seeking approval. This enables generic manufacturers to produce drugs more cheaply and is part of the reason why generics can provide cost savings. The threshold for bioequivalence in China is for the generic drug to reach blood concentrations of within 80–125% of the reference product, the same standard as used by the US FDA (Liao et al., 2015). Unfortunately, the largest gap in bioequivalence testing in China has been the lack of a unique reference product against which to test (as would be found in the US FDA's Orange Book). Bioequivalence testing of generics compared with off-patent originators has demonstrated significant differences in dissolution profiles (Hu et al., 2015).

Concerns about poor generic quality are not immaterial, as there have been high-profile lapses in the quality of domestically produced products (US-China Economic and Security Review Commission, 2014). Problems with drug quality have led to the creation of a large market for expensive off-patent originators produced by multinational corporations

(Boston Consulting Group, 2014). Surveys have shown off-patent originators can be up to 10 to 20 times the price of domestically produced generic competitors (Jiang et al., 2013, 2014; Wang et al., 2014a). A large survey of Chinese drug prices between 2002 and 2011 found that there was a consistent 40% average price gap between off-patent originators and domestic generics (Hu et al., 2015). Consequently, low domestic drug quality has driven demand for high-quality originator drugs from multinational corporations, leading to increases in average drug prices.

Raising the overall quality of domestic drugs in China can lead to higher use of lower priced generics, increasing access to medicines and decreasing OOP payments and THE. Many pricing policies are intended to narrow the often large gaps in price between off-patent branded originators and generics, but doing so requires that the generics be of the same quality as the branded originators and imported drugs. Various supply and demand-side policies have been used in the international setting to promote generics uptake, but doing so requires stronger regulations to guide quality (Sun, 2013).

The 2015 State Council Amendment has called for bioequivalence testing against a reference compound – either a reference listed drug or an internationally recognized drug – to be decided by an expert panel (State Council, 2015c). The government has also set a target of having all essential medications to be bioequivalent to reference products by 2018, with other drugs to follow afterwards. Drugs that fail bioequivalence testing will lose their market authorization. As there are hundreds of thousands of approved drugs with market authorization, ensuring they all comply with new bioequivalence standards will be a monumental task that will require significant investment in drug regulatory authorities. All of these measures should hopefully begin to narrow the gap, both real and perceived, between generics and their off-patent originators.

8.2.3 Challenges to foreign export

Drug quality is of particular concern when pharmaceutical companies try to export their products and are faced with international product standard regulations. Currently, Chinese GMP standards are not harmonized with international standards. Nevertheless, in the last few years, exports have been increasing substantially. For example, in the United States between 2007 and 2012, US FDA-regulated products from China increased from 1.3 million entry lines to 4.5 million (of which 67% were drugs and medical devices) (Van Arnum, 2013). The US FDA is charged with regulating quality of all pharmaceuticals distributed in the United States but has been struggling to complete inspections. In 2007, only 13 of 714 Chinese exporters to the United States were inspected (compared with 65 of 410 in India). The US FDA has had difficulties conducting inspections because of language barriers and also because inspectors cannot arrive unannounced as is their practice in the United States. Additionally, should they require extra time for an inspection it is difficult for them to extend their inspections because of tight itineraries (Vincent, 2014). United States-based drug manufacturers perceive the asymmetrical inspection process as unfair as they are subject to considerably more frequent, and in some ways more rigorous, US FDA inspections.

Problems with Chinese drug quality is increasingly recognized by the American public and this could affect the export capacity of Chinese manufacturing firms. One paper notes that "without proper inspection or oversight of foreign companies, the potential of adulterated products entering the United States or European markets is an accident waiting to happen" (Vincent, 2014). High-profile cases of lapses in drug quality, such as a counterfeit ingredient used in the production of an anticoagulant, which led to dozens of deaths, have increased both domestic and international concerns about Chinese drug quality (Edney, 2014).

US FDA and European Medicines Agency requirements will put increasing pressure on Chinese manufacturers to maintain GMP, especially as they hope to grow into foreign markets. The US FDA and the CFDA have been cooperating to increase regulation and inspection. For example, teams from both agencies have observed inspections by the other. Additionally, the CFDA provided the US FDA with a list of manufacturers who had action taken against them based on regulatory concerns (Van Arnum, 2013). Inter-institutional cooperation such as this will be a key component of maintaining the confidence of export markets. Even so, the US FDA still only has two permanent drug inspectors in its Beijing office and foreign counties must rely on China's own regulatory bodies (BloombergBusiness, 2015).

In order to be more competitive internationally and domestically, Chinese manufacturers must strengthen their GMP standards and eventually move towards international harmonization. Quality is of utmost concern when it comes to pharmaceuticals, and even a few lapses can generate significant mistrust and a shift away from domestic generic manufacturers to expensive imported medications. On an industrial policy level, increasing market concentration will help with this as a smaller number of larger companies should be easier to inspect and overall quality should increase.

8.3 Fragmentation of drug manufacturers

During the Communist era, drug manufacturing was centrally planned by the government (Dong et al., 1999). Since decentralization of production quotas, there has been a huge proliferation of drug manufacturers (Yu et al., 2010). According to the Chinese *National Health Statistics Handbook*, in 2011 China had 4629 drug manufacturers with an overall market concentration far lower than developed country peers. For example, the top five manufacturers hold only 13.2% of the total market share (IBISWorld, 2015c). This has led to dozens, and sometimes hundreds, of manufacturers seeking approval for an identical drug molecule, placing excessive burden on the CFDA. The government has been encouraging consolidation in recent years, recognizing the problems that market fragmentation can bring. As a result, the number of firms has been gradually declining, likely through acquisitions and mergers of manufacturing companies. Even so, fragmentation remains a huge concern.

This fragmentation has several effects. First, the regulatory burden on the CFDA is extraordinarily high, meaning that many drugs wait a long time for approval and Chinese patients then face delays in accessing the benefits of new medicines. Also, the volume of regulatory responsibility faced by the CFDA hinders its ability to perform adequate inspections, exacerbating issues caused by low quality standards. Fragmentation also supports the existence of low-cost manufacturers who subsist on bypassing quality standards, such as the API manufacturers who are less heavily regulated, potentially compromising pharmaceutical safety downstream. Finally, excessive fragmentation makes assembling the capacity for effective R&D difficult. Increasing market concentration should help to improve quality and is a government priority, but doing so is challenging because of protectionism at local and regional levels (Development Research Center of the State Council, 2015).

8.4 Fragmentation of drug distribution

The distribution network of Chinese pharmaceuticals is as fragmented as the manufacturing side. In China, there are over 13 853 drug wholesalers (compared with around 75 in the United States and 147 in Japan) (Center for Health Statistics and Information, 2013; Tse et al., 2012). In contrast to developed markets in the United States and Japan, where the top three distributors control 85% and 74% of market share, respectively, the top three Chinese distributors have only a 22% market share (Fig. 8.1) (Tse et al., 2012). Similar to manufacturers, distributors are also required to adhere to Good Supply Practice requirements. However, these licences can be difficult to acquire and require a high capital cost for both the licence and associated capital resources (e.g. equipment and facilities in compliance with regulation) (Ngai, 2014).

Fig. 8.1 Market share of the top three distributors for selected countries, 2008–2010

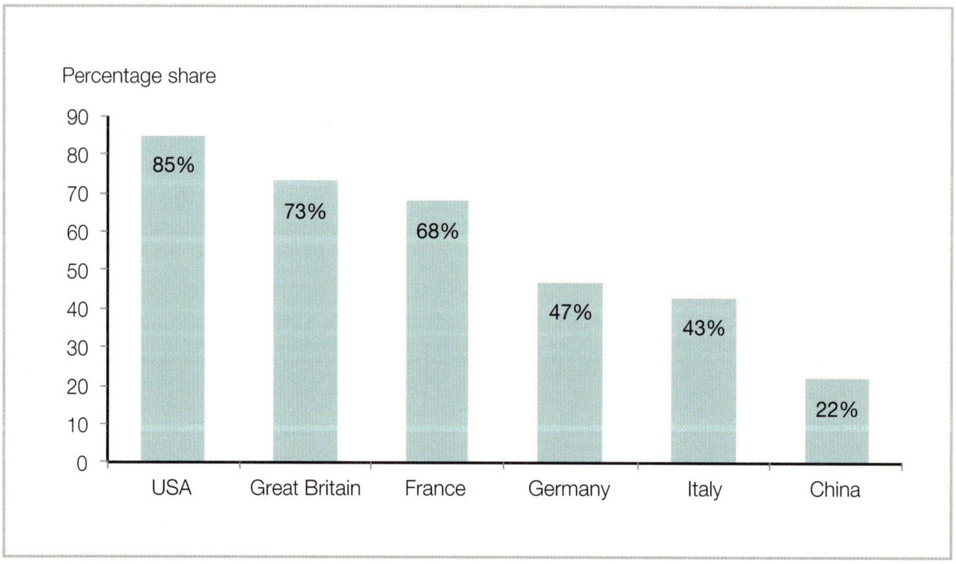

Source: Tse et al., 2012.

Geographic segmentation has been hard to overcome. Logistical challenges concerning transport across a large national territory are a significant barrier (Tse et al., 2012). Additionally, regional protectionism of local markets affects expansion and consolidation, such protectionism occurring in the form of requiring local business registration or restricting geographic distribution of drugs after centralized procurement (Institute of Economic Research, 2014).

Despite this, a few key players are emerging as distribution leaders. They tend to have developed from different geographical areas, and their market share is strongest in their particular regions. For example, Shanghai Pharma is based around the coastal cities, while Guangzhou Medicine Company is based around the southern cities. A few companies, such as SinoPharm and Jointown Pharma, have national networks (Tse et al., 2012). However, partly because of the fragmentation and varied payment processes, there can be a significant lag in payment time from the hospital to the distributor. This can put excessive strain on companies, especially on smaller ones that have difficulty surviving on intermittent capital flows (Tse et al., 2012).

The major distributors are embarking on strategies of consolidation through mergers and acquisitions. In this phase, they are concentrating on expanding market access to increase their national coverage. However, this will leave them with significant heterogeneity in operating processes among their acquired companies. Postmerger streamlining and standardization of these processes will be a significant challenge for these distributors (Tse et al., 2012). Government consolidation goals have been set in recognition of the potential efficiencies to be gained in this area, with the aim of having one to three national drug distributors with a turnover of RMB 100 billion, 20 with turnover of RMB 10 billion, and for the top 100 wholesalers to account for 85% of the market (Ngai, 2014).

8.5 Distribution and supply chains

There are several ways for a drug to reach a patient from the manufacturer. These may include any combination of distributors, pharmacies and hospitals along the way (Institute of Economic Research, 2014):

manufacturer → patient

manufacturer → hospital → patient

manufacturer → wholesaler → patient

manufacturer → pharmacy → patient

manufacturer → wholesaler → hospital → patient

manufacturer → wholesaler → pharmacy → patient.

In practice, approximately 80% of sales are through the pathway from manufacturer through wholesaler, hospital and to patient. In China, 70–80% of drug sales to the patient are through the hospital (Institute of Economic Research, 2014) in contrast to approximately 20% in developed countries (Lopez Bastida & Mossialos, 2000; Mossialos & Oliver, 2005; Tordoff, Norris & Reith, 2008). This is driven by the fact that drug sales are a major mechanism of hospital financing in China, although newer reforms aim to change this (Yu et al., 2010). Sales to hospitals are also bolstered by aggressive promotion from manufacturers to hospitals and prescribing physicians. Sales commissions and gifts to hospital managers and physicians create incentives to prescribe a particular manufacturer's product (Yu et al., 2010).

One problem with China's convoluted distribution system is the mark-ups that wholesalers and middlemen are able to charge along the chain. Anecdotally, the existence of multiple intermediaries often means the price patients pay can be up to ten times higher than the ex-factory price (Development Research Center of the State Council, 2015). An analysis by the health consultancy IMS Health estimates the average total mark-up between ex-factory and hospital price to be 52% (IMS Health, 2015b). These supply chain mark-ups contribute to the very high drug prices that patients end up facing.

8.6 Retail pharmacies

As with wholesalers, there has been a proliferation of retail pharmacies, with over 426 000 outlets as of 2011 (Center for Health Statistics and Information, 2013). In spite of the large numbers of retail pharmacies, they account for a relatively small proportion of total drug sales (Fig. 8.2) (Tse et al., 2012). Needless to say, fragmentation abounds also in this sector: in 2010, the top pharmacy companies only captured 22% of the market (Tse et al., 2012). The distribution model of some manufacturers (e.g. Jointown) is specifically to try to increase marketing to pharmacies (Tse et al., 2012). This may reduce the number of pharmacy chains and have positive effects on price and access, especially in geographically

Fig. 8.2 Evolution of pharmaceutical sales in China by channel, 2005–2015

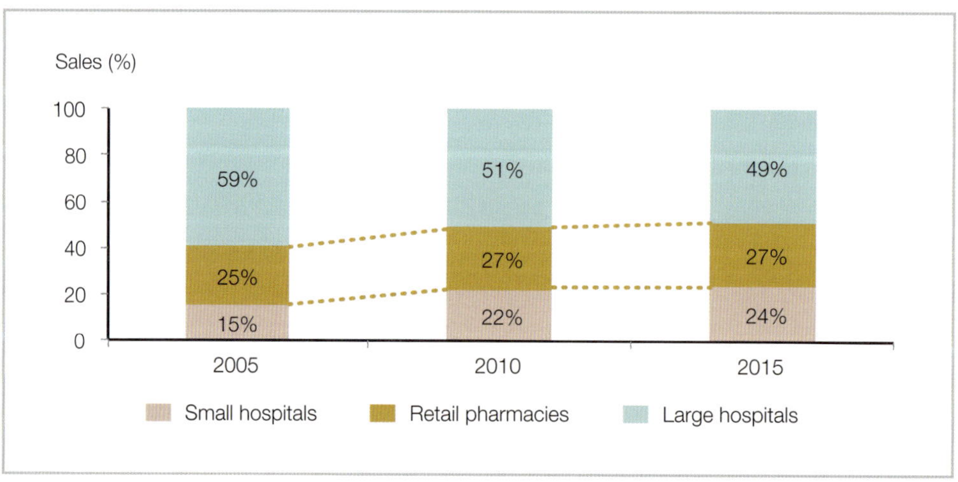

Source: Institute of Economic Research, 2014.

distant areas. Consolidation among pharmacies is also an official government target, with a goal of 60% market coverage by the top 100 drug retailers by 2015 (Ngai, 2014).

8.7 Conclusions

In recent years, there has been tremendous growth in the number pharmaceutical manufacturers, distributors and pharmacies in China. While this has enabled increased access to medicines in the health system, the rapid expansion has also introduced a number of difficulties throughout the supply chain. The CFDA is the national agency responsible for drug approval and quality, and it has been overwhelmed by the sheer number of drugs needing approval and guarantee of quality. Rapid expansion has led to inconsistent application of GMP and has challenged the ability to maintain high-quality inspection of manufacturers by both domestic and foreign agencies. The fragmentation of manufacturing has contributed to high-profile quality lapses and low consumer trust in pharmaceutical quality. Quality problems pose a risk to China's desire to export more medications and can raise concerns for foreign regulators. Recent policy announcements have aimed to improve the overall level of quality of the pharmaceutical market by targeting both the approvals process and drug quality standards.

Fragmentation along the supply chain means there are many ways for a drug to reach a consumer, with varying effects on price and reliable access. The presence of multiple intermediaries drives up prices for patients at the end of the supply chain. Additionally, there can be wide geographic variation in access and difficulties with supply chain logistics. A strategy of consolidation throughout the supply chain is ongoing and will help to remedy fragmentation issues and reduce the number of wholesalers who take mark-ups along the supply chain.

Unfortunately, increasing market concentration is difficult because of the extent to which local protectionism exists. Ultimately, China must strengthen the capacity of the CFDA, gradually move towards internationally harmonized standards for GMP and Good Supply Practice and engage in further consolidation of manufacturers and distributors to ensure that drugs are effective and safe for domestic and foreign use.

9. Irrational prescribing

KEY MESSAGES

- Irrational prescribing is endemic within the Chinese health care system. It is driven by perverse supply-side economic incentives such as the 15% mark-up policy as well as by demand-side factors such as incorrect beliefs about the efficacy of antibiotics and injections.
- The overprescribing and inappropriate prescribing of antibiotics and injections are particularly prominent:
  - approximately half of all antibiotics are prescribed inappropriately, with the average Chinese citizen consuming 138 g of antibiotics a year, ten times higher than in the United States; and
  - in some regions of China, more than half of prescriptions include an injection, far in excess of WHO recommendations of only about 13–24%.
- Irrational prescribing has significant negative consequences, such as a rapid increase in antimicrobial resistance and adverse drug reactions.
- Promoting medication adherence and preventing drug–drug and drug–herb interactions are also important components of rational prescribing that can be supported through better education on prescribing and the use of clinical decision-support tools.
- The EDL has had limited success in promoting the rationalization of prescribing at a primary care level. However, national campaigns aimed at rational prescribing in a hospital setting have had greater success.

9.1 Financial incentives and irrational prescribing

Irrational prescribing is a global problem, but one that is particularly serious in China because of the financial incentives that have caused pharmaceutical sales to become the major source of revenue for health care providers (Currie, Lin & Meng, 2014; Li et al., 2012; Zhang, 2010). From the 1980s onwards, health care facilities were allowed to charge a 15% mark-up on the sale of medications. Many hospitals encouraged aggressive drug sales by tying physician income to bonus payments that depended on the volume and value of drugs sold (Chen et al., 2014; Wagstaff et al., 2009).

The government is currently trying to remove the perverse prescribing incentive through policies such as ZMU and alternative payment mechanisms, but the legacy of over-prescribing is difficult to erase. Inappropriate prescribing by physicians has fuelled an incorrect belief that drugs are necessary for a number of conditions for which they are not medically indicated (Reynolds & McKee, 2011). This has created a vicious cycle of irrational prescribing driven by both physician incentive and patient demand.

9.2 Irrational prescribing of antibiotics and injections

Antibiotic overprescribing is a well-known problem, with China consuming about half of all the world's antibiotics (Zhang Q-Q et al., 2015). A study examining a large nationally representative sample of prescriptions written between 2007 and 2009 showed that patients at urban primary care institutions were prescribed on average 2.6 drugs per visit, which is nearly one more drug than recommended by the WHO (Li et al., 2012). In particular, antibiotics were prescribed nearly twice as much as recommended by the WHO. Several other studies also found excessive prescriptions of antibiotics (Dong, Yan & Wang, 2011; Jiang et al., 2012; Wang J et al., 2014; Yang et al., 2012; Yip et al., 2014). In general, it is estimated that about half of the antibiotics prescribed in China were medically unnecessary (Dong, Yan & Wang, 2011; Mao et al., 2015; Sun et al., 2008). A recent systematic review of the literature found that the median percentage of antibiotics prescribed per 100 encounters was 52.60% (Table 9.1) (Mao et al., 2015). On average, each Chinese individual consumes 138 g of antibiotics a year, 10 times the amount consumed in the United States (Li, 2014). Antibiotics are commonly used to treat viral infections such as upper respiratory tract infections for which they have no effect. (Li et al., 2012; Li, 2014; Yip et al., 2014). For example, it is estimated that about 75% of patients with viral influenza are prescribed antibiotics (Heddini et al., 2009).

Table 9.1 Key indicators of irrational prescribing in China

Prescribing indicator	
Number of medicines per prescription	2.94
Percentage of antibiotics per 100 encounters	52.60
Average number of antibiotics per encounter	0.75
Percentage of injections prescribed per 100 encounters	40.75

Source: Mao et al., 2015.

Antibiotics are also used extensively in livestock in China. More than half of China's antibiotics are used on animals (84 240 tons versus 77 760 tons in humans) (Zhang Q-Q et al., 2015). A recent study demonstrated that antibiotic overuse is so extensive that there are high concentrations of commonly used antibiotics throughout many of China's rivers, particularly in the eastern developed provinces (Zhang Q-Q et al., 2015).

Many of the studies investigating prescribing patterns in China have also reported overuse of injections. In one study of 10 rural provinces in China, it was found that excessive prescription of injections was actually the most prominent manifestation of irrational prescribing, more so even than that of antibiotics (Dong, Yan & Wang, 2011). Another study reported that the proportion of prescriptions with injections in Sichuan, a rural province, was 51.4% – far higher than the WHO recommendation of 13.4–24.1% for developing countries (Jiang et al., 2012). A systematic review found that the median percentage of injections prescribed per 100 encounters in China was 40.75% (Table 9.1) (Mao et al., 2015). As with antibiotics, injections, including the use of intravenous fluids, are commonly used inappropriately for conditions such as benign viral infections.

9.3 Drivers of irrational prescribing

There are a series of factors that explain the irrational prescribing patterns of antibiotics and injections outlined above. On the demand side, patients themselves frequently ask for antibiotics irrespective of need because of a common belief among Chinese citizens that antibiotics are a panacea (Li, 2014; Xiao et al., 2013). A survey of rural Chinese residents revealed that 62% of parents gave their children antibiotics without consulting a physician (Yu et al., 2014). This self-medication is made possible by the extensive practice of pharmacies selling antibiotics even without prescriptions (Fang, 2014). Furthermore, some patients believe that newer antibiotics are better and more effective, when in reality they often are no better (Li, 2014).

Similarly, popular belief in China holds that injections are more effective than oral medications (Jiang et al., 2012). This is coupled with the fact that the lay population generally lacks knowledge about the adverse consequences of overprescription, such as antimicrobial resistance and infections from injections (Li et al., 2012; Mao et al., 2015). Some doctors have admitted to prescribing antibiotics and injections upon request to please their patients as patients are free to choose their medical providers (Dong et al., 1999; Mao et al., 2015).

On the supply side, the Chinese Government directly subsidizes less than 10% of the operating costs of hospitals, leading them to seek other sources of funding (Li, 2014). Drug sales account for over 50% of all hospital revenues in many places, with antibiotics specifically contributing to up to 47% of drug sales (Li, 2014). As mentioned above, many hospitals link physician income and bonuses with meeting certain prescription quotas (Currie, Lin & Zhang, 2011). This and the 15% mark-up contribute to a powerful incentive for physicians to overprescribe. The retrospective fee-for-service payment methods commonly adopted in China for providers can exacerbate these perverse incentives to inappropriately prescribe as income is driven by quantity rather than quality of service provided (Chen et al., 2014). Taken together, this combination of supply-side and demand-side factors creates a powerful push towards overprescribing. A list of nine influential factors that were mentioned in a systematic review of irrational prescribing is presented in Table 9.2 (Mao et al., 2015).

Table 9.2 Influential factors driving irrational prescribing

Influential factors	No. (%) China (n = 67)
Health care providers' lack of skills and knowledge	9 (13.4%)
Patients' lack of knowledge	14 (20.9%)
Poor quality of health services	2 (3.0%)
Health facility's inadequate human resources and lack of qualified medical staff	–
Pressure from heavy patient load	2 (3.0%)
Pressure from patient demands	1 (1.5%)
Economic incentive and profits from prescribing medicines	20 (30.0%)
Insurance status of patients	4 (6.0%)
Lack of effective control and regulatory mechanisms on medicine use	3 (4.5%)

Source: Mao et al., 2015.

9.4 Adverse consequences of irrational prescribing

One of the reasons irrational prescribing of antibiotics is undesirable is because it can lead to adverse drug reactions and allergic responses (Yang et al., 2012). In China, some 2.5 million patients are admitted to hospitals each year as a result of serious adverse drug events. For example, 60% of all children with acquired deafness developed the condition through irrational use of ototoxic drugs (Yang et al., 2012).

Irrational prescribing also causes antibiotic resistance, where a microorganism develops resistance to an antimicrobial drug that was originally effective for its treatment. There is a consequent loss in the range of effective drugs to fight infections, as well as increased health care costs, prolonged hospitalization and substantially increased social and economic burden (Wang J et al., 2014). The morbidity and mortality from infections caused by multidrug-resistant pathogens are higher in China than in many other countries (Xiao et al., 2013; Yezli & Li, 2012). In fact, China now has the world's most rapid growth rate of resistance as a result of antibiotics abuse. In particular, the prevalence of hospital "superbugs" such as extended spectrum beta-lactamase-producing *Escherichia coli* and methicillin-resistant *Staphylococcus aureus* are significantly increasing in tertiary hospitals under China's heavy antibiotic environment (Li, 2014). Recently, Chinese animals were found to harbour bacteria containing a gene that conferred resistance to polymyxins and could easily be transferred to other bacteria (Liu et al., 2015). This is particularly concerning as polymyxins were the last class of antibiotics in which resistance could not easily be spread from bacteria to bacteria.

The overuse of injections can also be hazardous as there is a risk of unsafe needles leading to infection or transmission of blood-borne infections such as hepatitis B and C or HIV/AIDS (Dong, Yan & Wang, 2011; Song et al., 2014b). Furthermore, injections are more expensive than comparative oral drug therapies because of the additional cost of syringes, sterilization control and well-trained personnel (Song et al., 2014b).

High levels of irrational drug prescribing also drives higher volumes of drug sales, which increases overall health expenditure. While it is unclear what proportion of China's pharmaceutical expenditure comes from irrational prescribing, it is likely to be a significant amount. Irrational prescribing can, therefore, increase health care spending through both direct drug costs and the indirect costs associated with dealing with adverse reactions and antibiotic resistance.

9.5 Adherence and drug interactions

Medication adherence and drug interactions are two other key aspects of rational prescribing. Adherence is particularly important for chronic diseases, which require patients to take medicines up to several times a day for the rest of their lives. It is estimated that up to 50% of patients do not take their medicines as prescribed (Brown & Bussell, 2011). Drug–drug interactions and drug–herb interactions (between western drugs and TCM preparations) pose substantial health risks to patients, particularly in the context of general overprescribing. An Institute of Medicine report from the United States estimated that around 7000 people die annually from medication errors (Institute of Medicine, 2000). Other studies estimated that drug interactions accounted for 3–5% of all in-hospital medication errors and were an important cause of patient visits to emergency departments (Leape et al., 1995; Raschetti et al., 1999).

There is a significant body of anecdotal research that suggests that medication adherence is also a problem in China. Studies have assessed that compliance with treatment of chronic diseases such as hypertension and diabetes can be quite low, in the 50–60% range (Lee et al., 2013; Wang W et al., 2014; Xin et al., 2015; Zhang Y et al., 2015). Compliance was even lower among patients with schizophrenia, with 12-month continuation rates as low as 10% (Yao et al., 2013). Migrants were also found to have low compliance rates for tuberculosis treatment (Tang et al., 2015). Poor adherence is harmful to patients themselves and, in the case of highly contagious diseases such as tuberculosis, to the general public. There are many ways in which prescription adherence can be improved. These include patient education, minimizing pill burden, letting patients know about side-effects ahead of time, and better communication between hospitals and primary care.

The likelihood of drug interactions is increasing as more medicines are used in China. For example, warfarin, a commonly used anticoagulant, is known to interact with a number of antibiotics. Chinese patients are particularly at risk given the large amounts of antibiotics that are prescribed. Another area of concern is drug–herb interactions. Some of these include bleeding when warfarin is combined with gingko or dong quai, serotonin syndrome in patients using St John's Wort with antidepressants, and decreased concentrations of prednisolone when taken with the herbal product Xiao chai hu tang (Fugh-Berman, 2000). Unfortunately, the mechanism of action of many TCMs are not understood so interactions are challenging to predict. In addition to provider and patient education, one of the key strategies in reducing drug interactions is the use of clinical decision-support system, such as electronic medical records, which provide drug interaction warnings (Institute of Medicine, 2006). Unfortunately, such electronic systems are not commonly used throughout China and capacity will have to be gradually built.

9.6 Policies to combat irrational prescribing in China

China's EDL was launched in 2009 partly to combat the irrational prescribing patterns plaguing primary care facilities and county hospitals (Chen, 2009). The EDL was introduced in conjunction with the ZMU policy, in which health care facilities would no longer be allowed to charge the 15% mark-up. The EDL was initially implemented in primary care facilities and is gradually being expanded to hospitals. From the perspective of rationalizing prescription use, the EDL was not as successful as hoped. Most studies have looked at the role of the EDL at the level of primary care as this is where it was first introduced. Results indicate that, while there are sometimes small decreases in the amount of irrationally prescribed antibiotics or injections, overall levels of prescribing remain high and far in excess of WHO standards (Song et al., 2014b; Xiang et al., 2012; Yang et al., 2012).

There have been several antibiotic containment campaigns aimed at hospitals that have been more successful. In 2011, the Chinese Government launched a national antibiotic stewardship campaign against the overuse of antibiotics with an action plan that was compulsory for class II and III hospitals (Bao et al., 2015; Tao et al., 2013). The protocol consisted of establishing mandatory administrative strategies for the rational use of antimicrobial drugs, setting targets for antimicrobial management, organizing task forces, developing audit and inspection systems and investigating and reassigning responsibility from management staff who violated rational prescribing (Xiao et al., 2013). Hospitals that failed to meet targets were downgraded to a lower classification level and hospital leadership could even potentially be dismissed. Medical personnel who seriously violated regulations could lose the accreditation needed to prescribe antibiotics and other drugs, have their professional qualification revoked or even be criminally prosecuted in extreme situations. Directors of hospital departments were to hold weekly meetings to discuss issues pertaining to antibiotic administration, and health care authorities conducted two supervision sessions each year during which the hospital's performance relating to antibiotics was inspected (Bao et al., 2015; Tao et al., 2013).

In March 2012, the government initiated the Circular for Further Promotion of the Regulation on Antibiotics Prescription in Hospitals to strengthen the supervision of antibiotics use in county public hospitals (Tao et al., 2013). In May of the same year, the Management Provision for Clinical Application of Antibiotics was introduced. This document established guidelines that were intended to further regulate and restrict the undesired antibiotic-prescribing behaviours of physicians and to encourage prescribing on the basis of comprehensive physical examination and laboratory investigations (Li, 2014; Tao et al., 2013). Furthermore, only 50 and 35 antibiotic agents, respectively, were to be made available to city and county hospitals (Xiao et al., 2013). In addition, antibiotics would be classified into three categories on the basis of effectiveness, clinical safety, side-effect profile and price: non-limited (first line), limited (second line) and specifically controlled (third line) (Tao et al., 2013). First-line antibiotics (high effectiveness and safety, low price and few side-effects) were recommended as the first-choice agent while use of second- and third-line antibiotics was generally discouraged unless necessary. Other policies that have shown promise in hospitals include the introduction of electronic medical records as well as accreditation to international standards for antimicrobial stewardship (Li J-S et al., 2013; Song, Li & Zhou, 2014). As of 2015, there were some 20 national programmes and policies instituted for rationalizing antibiotic prescribing in the areas of human resources capacity-building, clinical guidelines, surveillance, prescription reform and health care provider education (Xiao & Li, 2015).

Between 2011 and 2014, antibiotic prescribing rates fell from 62.9% to 35.3% in an inpatient setting and from 26.4% to 12.9% in an outpatient setting in 65 sampled hospitals, which is a success given that the goals set by the action plan were 60% and 20% reductions (Bao et al., 2015). The same study reported significant reductions in patient spending on antibiotics as well. Other studies report similar declines in antibiotic use. National surveillance data showed success in a number of areas, including decreased use of antibiotics in surgical procedures and in the use of treatment with two or more antibiotics (Xiao & Li, 2015). IMS Health data showed that antibiotics made up 17% of the total value of hospital drug sales in the fourth quarter of 2012, down from 25% in 2011 (Xiao et al., 2013). Another evaluation of 420 hospitals demonstrated a decline in overall antibiotic sales growth from 31.64% in the first quarter of 2010 to -23.46% in the fourth quarter of 2011 (Fig. 9.1) (Tao et al., 2013). Segmenting antibiotic sales by class, an increase in the use of first-line antibiotics and a decrease in the use of second- and third-line antibiotics has also been observed (Fig. 9.2) (Tao et al., 2013).

Fig. 9.1 Growth of sales value for antibiotics in selected hospitals, 2010 and 2011

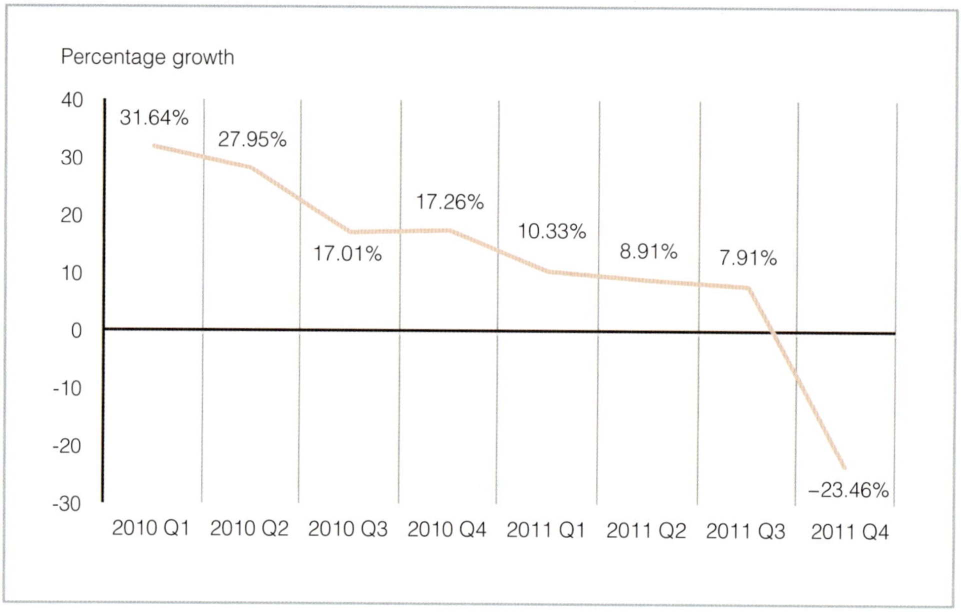

Source: Tao et al., 2013.

Note: Q1–Q4: Quarters 1–4.

Fig. 9.2 **Sale value growth and volume growth for first-line (a), second-line (b) and third-line (c) antibiotics in selected hospitals for 2010 and 2011**

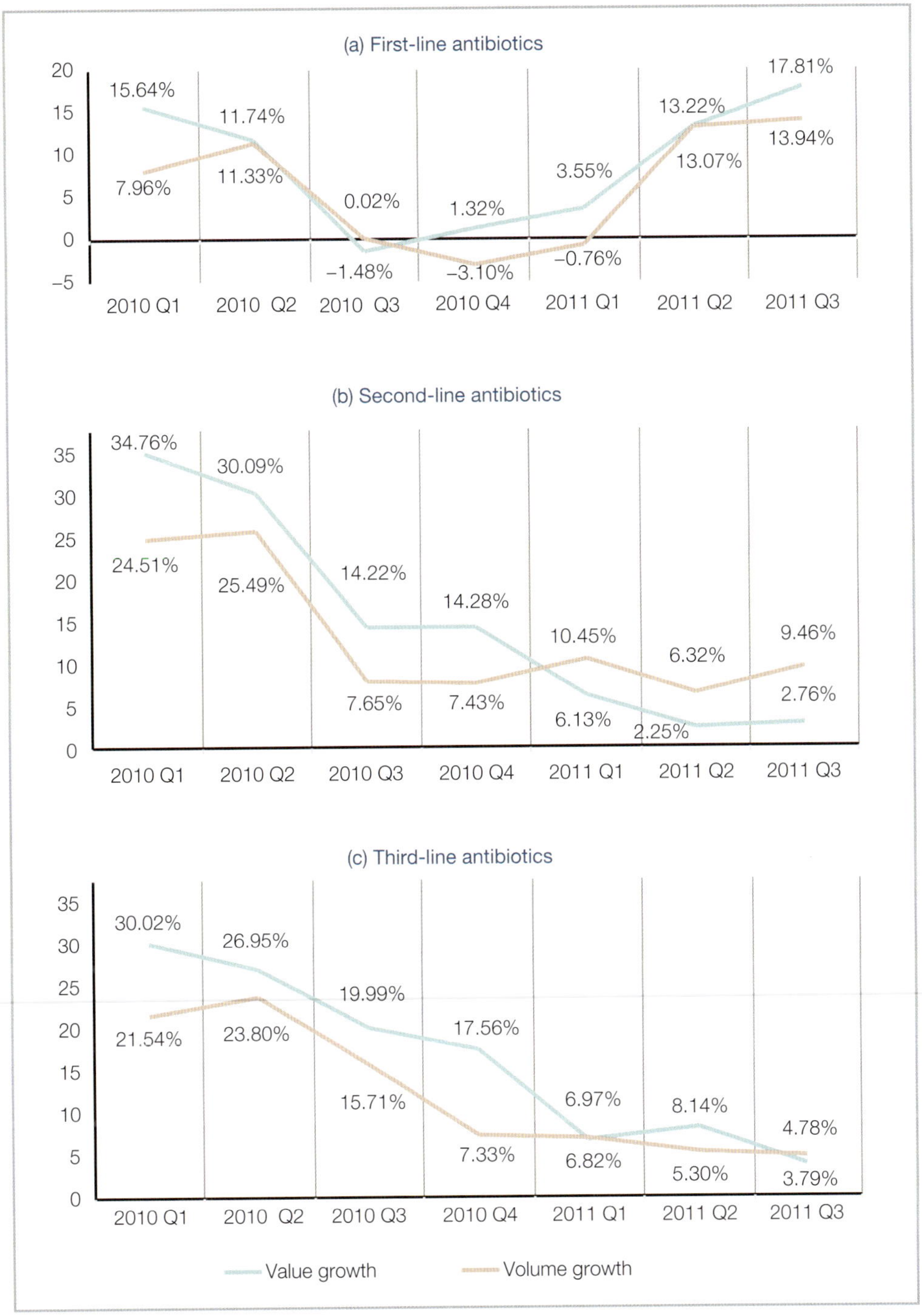

Source: Tao et al., 2013.

Note: Q1–Q4: Quarters 1–4.

9.7 Conclusions

Irrational prescribing is a huge problem in China's health care system, with rates of antibiotic and injection use far in excess of WHO guidelines. This has been driven by a combination of supply-side policies – largely an incentive to overprescribe to generate income – and demand-side issues, with patients frequently demanding inappropriate medications. The epidemic of irrational prescribing has driven up rates of antimicrobial resistance and adverse drug events.

Recently, efforts have been made to reverse the problem of irrational prescribing. At the primary care level, the EDL has sought to rationalize prescribing through the introduction of the ZMU policy to take away the incentive to sell more medications. It has had limited success in decreasing antibiotic and injection use. In hospitals, various national campaigns targeted at decreasing antibiotic use seem to have been more successful. Moving forwards, the ZMU will be implemented in more hospitals and hopefully will contribute to further declines in antibiotic and other irrational drug use. Improving medication adherence and limiting drug interactions are also crucial for rationalizing prescribing in China.

A comprehensive strategy to improve prescribing will improve health and decrease costs. Further roll-out of the ZMU policy, broader implementation of clinical practice guidelines and information systems and education campaigns for patients and providers will hopefully lead to further declines in irrational drug use. Electronic information systems will be particularly helpful not only in guiding rational prescribing through clinical reminders and order sets but also in conducting drug utilization reviews. However, any policies that seek to take away drug revenue from health care facilities will have to be initiated in tandem with increased government subsidies in order for them to be sustainable.

10. Hospitals and pharmaceutical policy

KEY MESSAGES

- China is heavily reliant on hospitals for the provision of health care services because of its weak primary care system. Hospitals account for about 65% of THE and between 70% and 80% of TPE.
- Drug sales form a large portion of hospital revenues (~40%), which encourages excessive and inefficient prescribing. A large portion of drug costs come from patients' OOP spending, which is harmful for access and equity.
- Public hospital reforms have sought to remove the link between hospital revenues and drug sales with the introduction of ZMU pilots. China has launched two rounds of urban hospital reforms and several rounds of county hospital reforms. The State Council has set an ambitious target of universal adoption of ZMU at all county hospitals by 2015 and all urban hospitals by 2017.
- While evidence for the effects of urban hospital reforms is relatively sparse, at the county level, ZMU has led to a decline in drug sales as a proportion of revenues.
- Severing the link between hospital revenue and drug sales will require alternative funding channels to be explored, primarily through adjustments in service fees or greater government subsidies. Otherwise, hospitals will be fiscally unsustainable.
- Hospital reforms have so far been largely devolved to local governments because of considerations of local context and funding capabilities. As a result, reforms have been piecemeal and their outcomes poorly reported.
- Private hospitals are being encouraged in order to introduce competition to challenge the current monopoly of public hospitals, with a target of 20% non-public service provision by 2015. However, caution must be taken to ensure that these entities do not prioritize profit-seeking behaviour.

10.1 Introduction to hospitals in China

Hospitals are the cornerstone of China's health care system. China has a very weak primary care system so is heavily reliant on its hospital system. In terms of health provision, hospitals deliver more than 90% of the country's inpatient services and a substantial portion of its outpatient services (Yip et al., 2012). Hospitals also account for about 65% of THE, a figure which has remained steady this century (Barber et al., 2014). In contrast, hospital spending in European countries account for only 20–40% of THE (Masseria et al., 2009). Hospitals also account for around 70–80% of all pharmaceutical sales in China (National Health Development Research Center, 2013), compared with only about 20–40% in OECD countries (OECD, 2015b). Given the importance of hospitals in China's health care system, public hospital reform was identified as one of the five pillars of China's 2009 health care reforms.

CHCs provide primary care in urban settings and THCs provide primary care in rural settings. Meanwhile, large general hospitals at city, provincial and national levels are responsible for treating more complicated diseases, engaging in research and training new physicians. In rural settings, primary care is provided by THCs and village clinics while county-level hospitals provide for more complex care. In 2011, China had 21 979 hospitals including 11 642 urban hospitals (2 220 287 beds) and 10 337 rural hospitals (1 484 831 beds). By ownership, 13 539 were public hospitals (3 243 658 beds) and 8440 were non-public hospitals (461 460 beds) (WHO & China National Health Development Research Center, 2012).

The network of hospitals is classified according to a three-tier system (primary, secondary or tertiary), with each tier further divided into three functional levels. Hospital tiers are based on a scoring system that ranks an institution's ability to provide medical care, medical education and conduct medical research. Considerations include the number and type of departments, human resources, number of beds and teaching and research capabilities. Functional subclassifications (A, B or C) divide hospitals according to technical performance, quality management and performance and level of technology. The highest designation is reserved for tertiary hospitals that are considered domestic leaders in their field and can exert international influence. This subset of tertiary hospitals is designated as A+ institutions (Ministry of Health, 1989).

According to the National Health Service System Plan (2015–2020) released by the NHFPC in 2014, China is planning to have 6 inpatient beds per 1000 people, allocated across different tiers of public and private hospitals (Table 10.1) (NHFPC, 2014a; State Council, 2015e). This compares to a current inpatient bed status of 4.55 per 1000 people.

Hospitals are managed mainly by the NHFPC, but various ministries have powers to decide on policies that affect the day-to-day operation of hospitals. For example, medical service fees are set by the NDRC, while human resources are regulated by the Ministry of Human Resources and Social Security. Consequently, public hospitals can face conflicting policies from the many ministries that govern them.

Table 10.1 NHFPC targets in health service infrastructure and resources, 2015–2020

Parameter	2020 target	2013 status	Nature of target
Inpatient hospital beds per 1 000 residents	6.00	4.55	Suggested
Hospitals	4.80	3.56	Suggested
Public hospitals	3.30	3.04	Binding
Private hospitals	1.50	0.52	Suggested
Community health clinics	1.20	0.99	Suggested
Number of registered physicians per 1 000 residents	2.50	2.06	Suggested
Number of registered nurses per 1 000 residents	3.14	2.05	Suggested
Number of registered public health personnel per 1 000 residents	0.83	0.61	Suggested
Number of general practitioners per 10 000 residents	2.00	1.07	Binding
Ratio of physicians to nurses	1:1.25	1:1	Suggested
Ratio of beds to nurses for hospitals at city level and above	1:0.60	1:0.45	Suggested
Number of beds at county-level general hospitals	500	–	Suggested
Number of hospital beds at city-level general hospitals	800	–	Suggested
Number of hospitals at province-level general hospitals	1 000	–	Suggested

Sources: NHFPC, 2014a; State Council, 2015e.

10.2 Pharmaceutical spending in hospitals

A series of economic reforms in the 1980s and 1990s granted hospitals the right to charge a 15% mark-up on sales of pharmaceutical products to compensate for low government prices for medical services. Low service fee schedules are a vestige of the early 1950s planned economy era, which set prices below cost to guarantee implicit universal access to health care. The revenue gap was made up by government subsidies, which amounted to 60% of hospital operating budgets before the economic reform era but was unsustainable in the posteconomic reform environment (Yip & Eggleston, 2004).

Consequently, hospitals grew reliant on sales of pharmaceutical products to fund day-to-day operations. Drug sales steadily made up about 40% of hospital budgets from 2006 to 2011, whereas various direct government subsidies amounted to only 7–8% (Fig. 10.1) (Barber et al., 2014; Center for Health Statistics and Information, 2013).

Fig. 10.1 Hospital budget breakdown according to income stream, 2006–2012

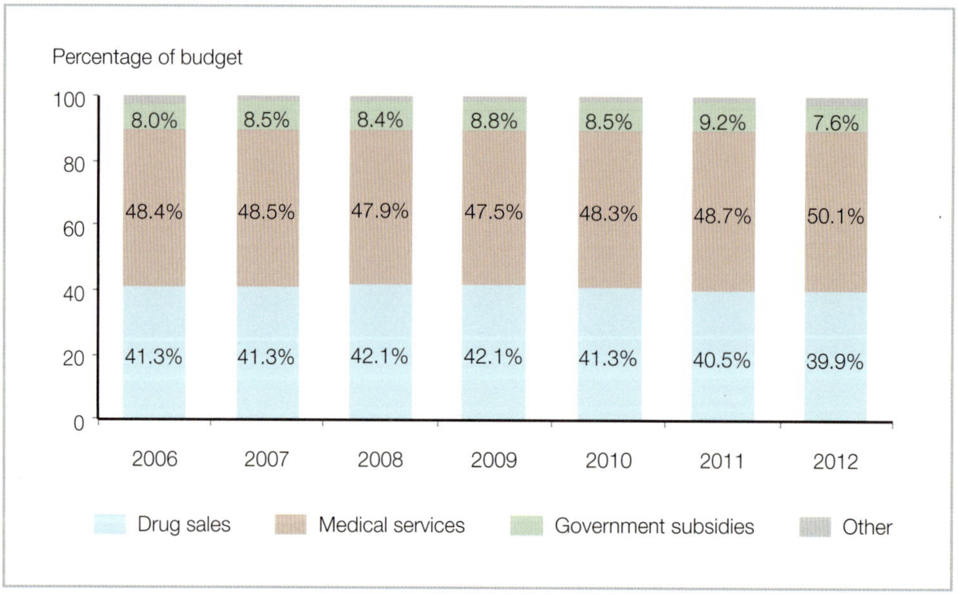

Sources: Barber et al., 2014; Center for Health Statistics and Information, 2013.

If segmented by source of funding, OOP funding forms the single largest source of public hospital revenue at 32%; various insurance schemes account for 60% of revenue, while direct government subsidies account for only 8% of revenue (Fig. 10.2) (McKinsey, 2010). The total government contribution to hospital revenues, even accounting for their contribution to insurance pools, is quite low at only 21% of total revenue.

Fig. 10.2 Breakdown of public hospital funding in China, 2010

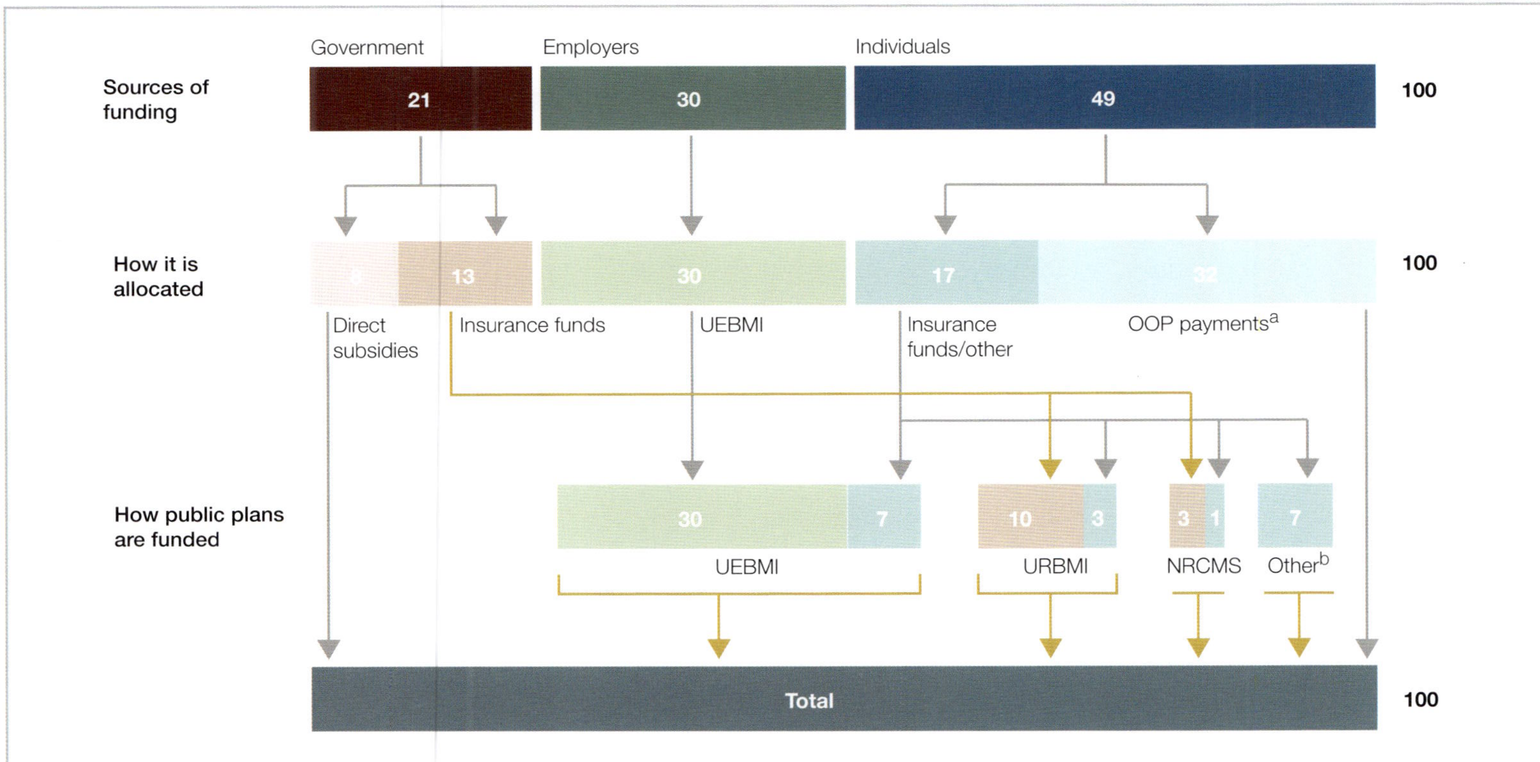

Source: McKinsey, 2010.

Notes: [a] Includes £6 million from the uninsured and $26 million in co-payments form the insured; b Total of ~£7 million and including private health insurance (supplementary and stand-alone) but not employer contribution to group private health insurance ($1 million);

NRCMS: New Rural Cooperative Medical Scheme.

Urban public hospitals are thought to be the core driver of pharmaceutical spending in China, accounting for 50% of growth through to 2020 (Boston Consulting Group, 2014). However, county hospitals are projected to be an increasingly important channel, given favourable government reimbursement policies and continued investment in infrastructure and training. Annual growth in drug spending at county hospitals will outpace growth in urban hospitals, retail pharmacies and primary care facilities (Boston Consulting Group, 2014).

10.3 Perverse incentives in hospitals

Historically, physicians and hospitals have had incentives to prescribe expensive and unnecessary treatments. This has been exacerbated by the fact that the majority of public hospitals are paid retrospectively via fee for service, where providers are not held financially accountable for the quality of service provided. Physicians working in public hospitals typically have low base salaries but are rewarded with large bonuses linked to overall hospital revenue, which is predominantly driven by sales of pharmaceutical products. As such, physicians have an incentive to prescribe according to profit margin rather than clinical efficacy. Pharmaceutical manufacturers have also moved in the form of kickbacks to capitalize on physician willingness to prescribe medicines to maximize profit. The United Kingdom-based pharmaceutical giant GlaxoSmithKline was fined RMB 3 billion (US$488 million) after a court in Hunan Province found the drug maker to have "offered money or property to non-government personnel in order to obtain improper commercial gains" (Ward, 2014). Kickbacks are so institutionalized that they have been estimated to account for more than 20% of a drug's final retail price (*The Economist*, 2014b).

The portrayal of doctors as profit-seeking villains has resulted in growing distrust between the medical profession and patients, which has escalated to new heights in recent years with many reports of violent attacks on medical workers by disgruntled patients. In 2010, more than 17 000 incidents of violence against hospital staff occurred in China (*The Economist*, 2012). A survey by the China Hospital Management Association found that violence against medical personnel rose an average of 23% each year between 2002 and 2012 (Tatlow, 2013). Tales of violent attacks on Chinese providers have not escaped international media attention, with the *Lancet* and the *New Yorker* both publishing commentary on the incidents (Beam, 2014; Lancet Editorial, 2012).

In addition, retail pharmacies, often an independent sector in other countries, have a limited role in China. Cost-containment policies of more mature markets often leverage the split between hospitals and pharmacies so as to align pharmacy incentives to dispense lower-cost generics. Such a split does not exist in China, with most hospitals owning their own pharmacies. Reasons underpinning the relatively weak dispensing power of retail pharmacies are rooted in the historical development of the sector, as well as the general belief that hospitals deliver services of higher quality. It is estimated that only 20% of prescription medications are dispensed from community pharmacies (Fang et al., 2013). The government is actively promoting the growth of retail pharmacies to prevent hospitals from selling drugs to raise revenue.

10.4 Public hospital reform pilots

Given the large role of public hospitals in China's health service delivery and in driving pharmaceutical spending, initiating public hospital reform pilots was one of the five pillars of the massive health care reform, launched by the State Council in 2009.

The first wave of public hospital reform consisted of 17 national and 37 provincial pilots. In the guidance issued jointly by five central government departments in late 2010, nine large reform objectives were outlined (Ministry of Health et al., 2010). The reform most salient to pharmaceutical policy was reforming the public hospital financing mechanisms. Essentially, the government wanted to remove the link between the sales of drugs and hospital revenues in order to remove the perverse incentives described above; this was the intention of the introduction of policies such as ZMU. In 2014, a second wave of national public urban hospital pilots was launched that designated an additional 17 cities (NHFPC, 2014b).

Aside from reform pilots in urban centres, reform pilots were also launched in public county hospitals even more extensively; 311 pilot counties were involved in the first wave of county-level reforms launched in 2012. In addition to these nationally designated reform counties, 454 counties voluntarily adopted ZMU. In 2014, the number of counties participating in public county hospital reform pilots was also expanded to a total of 1101 counties, representing over 50% of counties in China.

The most recent 2015 State Council work plan for hospital reform states that, by 2017, the ZMU policy will be introduced across all urban hospitals, drug revenue will only be able to account for 30% of hospital revenue and OOP spending may account for only 20% of hospital revenue. Given the facts that currently very few hospitals have introduced ZMU, drug revenues generally account for 40% of revenues and OOP spending makes up over 30% of revenues, these targets are quite ambitious. County-level hospital reforms have also been listed for universal implementation by the end of 2015 (State Council, 2015d).

10.5 Political challenges of hospital reform

There was widespread recognition of the difficulty of hospital reform prior to its implementation. This sentiment was echoed by Former Premier Wen Jiabao, who described public hospital reform as the toughest "hard bone" in the newest round of health care reform given the entrenched interests and inertia involved (He, 2011). Prior to the formal launch of the public hospital reform pilots, two major setbacks were experienced.

First, the NHFPC, which was mandated to take a leading role, promised to conclude national pilots in 2010 and leverage experience from successful pilots in 2011. This was undermined by the inability to reach a consensus among all involved ministries. Consequently, the national policy guidance for pilots was postponed at least twice and was not started until 2010. Second, the inability of ministries to agree on proposals resulted in general, rather than specific, guidance on critical aspects of the reform. The debate mainly centred on increased government subsidizes in lieu of abolishing drug mark-ups.

The NHFPC attempted to bargain for more funding in the face of potential large deficits once drug mark-ups were abolished. These proposals were questioned by more powerful ministries, particularly the Ministry of Finance, which was sceptical given the historical inefficiencies pervasive throughout the system (Development Research Center of the State Council, 2015). The lack of specific guidance meant that local governments were able to determine the size of the subsidy according to local fiscal capabilities.

10.6 Urban hospital reform: lack of high-quality assessment

To date, there remains no objective, independent, system-level assessment of the outcome of the urban hospital pilots (Barber et al., 2014). There are several potential reasons for the lack of quality assessments. First, the second wave of pilots was only started in 2014 so there has been little time for evaluation to occur. Second, the broad scope of the pilots made it difficult to summarize their impact at the systems level. Third, while the NHFPC issued general guidelines, local governments were allowed to proceed based on their own fiscal strength, insurance coverage levels and other socioeconomic conditions. Finally, the pilots themselves were extremely complex and involved many simultaneous changes, making evaluation challenging.

Renmin University's Health Reform and Development Centre published a policy implementation assessment (but not an outcomes assessment) of the first round of public urban hospital reform in 2013 (Hufeng, 2013). The objective of the study was to retrospectively assess the degree to which local pilots were compliant with requirements outlined by central guidance. The rationale for undertaking an implementation study, rather than an outcomes evaluation, was based on the belief that "outcomes should follow on the basis of a thorough understanding of what has been implemented" (Hufeng, 2013).

The study found that the part of the central government's guidance generally associated with service management was implemented successfully by a majority of nationally designated cities. Examples of this include enhancing the quality of medical service management, increasing government subsidies and improving hospital information systems. However, other policies related to institutional reform were not as successfully implemented. These included clearly defining responsibilities for all levels of government-owned hospitals and separation of hospital financing from drug sales.

The NHFPC also released a short summary outlining anecdotal evidence of implementation in urban public hospital reforms as achieved by individual pilot sites (Ministry of Health, 2011b). Some of the following highlights were noted:

- Beijing, Shanghai and Anshan local governments guaranteed government investment for new infrastructure and large medical equipment purchases in public hospitals;
- Beijing gave full protection to health care costs for retirees; Wuhu and Ma'anshan City used government subsidies to enrol all retirees into a social pension system;
- Beijing established cost-based government subsidies for public hospitals;

- Shaanxi Province transferred budgeting of county hospital employees under the mandate of the government and guaranteed full protection for the budgeted amount;
- Anshan City, Ma'anshan City and Shaanxi Province began to explore gradually resolving public hospitals' historic debt; and
- Anhui Province devolved the right to price medical service fees to pilot cities.

A recent announcement by the NHFPC, the Ministry of Finance and the State Council on an evaluation of urban hospital pilots hinted at mixed results in removing the over-prescribing incentive and decreasing patient costs (Wang, 2015). In spite of this lack of strong evidence, the State Council is committed to continuing their public hospital reforms and broadening them nationwide by 2017.

10.7 County hospital reform: successes and challenges

More objective assessments are available for county hospital reforms (NHFPC, 2013b). In terms of abolishing drug markets at pilot county-level hospitals, of the first 311 national government designated counties, 299 successfully introduced ZMU. Aside from nationally designated counties, an additional 454 counties voluntarily abolished drug mark-up. By the end of 2014, 66% of Chinese counties had abolished drug mark-ups. Lost revenue was made up through a combination of increasing service fees and increasing government subsidies. Most regions did choose to do both, but determining the ratio of increased funding from subsidies versus service charges was unclear. Government subsidies, while significantly increased, were still insufficient in many areas.

Government subsidies for county public hospital pilots was realized in three ways: subsidies for employee salaries and basic operations, subsidies according to service volume, and subsidies according to bed number. For example, Lufeng County in Yunnan Province offered a RMB 6000/bed per year standard subsidy, which increased total funding by RMB 2.362 million. Where the subsidies came from also varied by province: in Anhui the majority of subsidies were provided by the province, while in Henan the ratio of subsidies were 2:1:2 for province, city and county, respectively.

In aggregate, abolishment of drug mark-up in pilot county public hospitals resulted in a revenue deficit of RMB 4.509 billion, of which 53.7% (RMB 2.422 billion) was subsidized through service fee increases and 18.78% (RMB 0.892 billion) was subsidized through government subsidies. There remained an RMB 1.196 billion deficit that was internalized and significantly increased fiscal pressure. Overall, county public hospital reform has shown positive signs in removing the link between drug sales and revenues. In a subset of 38 public county hospitals participating in the pilot that introduced ZMU in 2011, total pharmaceutical sales revenue declined from 42.7% of hospital revenue in 2011 to 38.1% in 2012. Conversely, hospital service charges as a percentage of hospital revenue rose from 29.3% in 2011 to 45.6% in 2012. These statistics demonstrate that ZMU can indeed cause county hospitals' revenues to rely less on pharmaceutical sales, but they also highlight the need for government subsidies to make up for lost revenues.

10.8 Other hospital-based pharmaceutical reforms

Aside from pilots executed as part of the public hospital reform, other policy changes have sought to limit the number and types of drug hospitals can stock. In 2011, the NHFPC released "Tertiary General Hospital Evaluation Criteria", which issued guidance on performance assessments in six general areas: infrastructure, medical service, patient safety, medical service quality and safety management, quality assurance, and hospital management (Ministry of Health, 2011a). In this document, limits are placed on the number of EDL formulations by hospital type, with 500–800 bed hospitals limited to a maximum of 1000 western and 200 TCM drugs and hospitals with more than 800 beds limited to a maximum of 1200 western and 300 TCM drugs. By constraining the number of competing formulations and generics for any given EDL item, the government hopes to promote quality and cost-containment (Guangdong Provincial HFPC, 2012).

Similarly, the NHFPC released the "Hospital Prescription Review Management (Pilot)", a guidance meant to "improve prescription quality, promote rational drug use and protect the health and safety of the patient" (Ministry of Health, 2010). In the document, violation citations can be given for low use of EDL drugs without reason, ill-suited modes of administration, unreasonable use of high-priced drugs and prescriptions of two or more drugs with the same pharmacological effects. Physicians exceeding a certain number of citations within a review cycle can be subject to training, fines and other penalties.

Other countries have incorporated multifaceted strategies to improve prescribing. These include prescribing budgets in parts of the United Kingdom and Germany in conjunction with financial penalties for overprescribing compared with that of peers. As ZMU is more broadly implemented, such budgets could provide further incentive to limit costly or unnecessary prescribing.

10.9 Private hospitals in China

Private hospitals have always existed in China but have historically had a limited role in service provision. However, the new health care reforms aim to promote their growth. Since the 2009 State Council "Opinions of the CPC Central Committee and the State Council Regarding Deepening the Health Care Reform" to encourage private capital to invest in non-profit-making hospitals, the policy landscape surrounding private hospitals has drastically shifted. In 2011, the State Council released Notification 11 on "Issuing of Program and Implementation Plan of Deepening Health System Reform in the Period of the 12th Five Year Plan", which called for more foreign investment in private hospitals and to have 20% of bed volume and health services provided by non-public institutions by 2015 (State Council, 2012b). Reasons for the strong push towards increasing private provision include using private competition to encourage change in an often stagnant public sector an ideological shift towards a more pro-market approach and the ability to mobilize private sector wealth to increase overall funding (Yip & Hsiao, 2014).

Although the number of private health care institutions has grown tremendously in China since 2005, their combined service volume and equivalent value is still quite low. In 2005, 17% of hospitals were privately owned; this number has since increased to 42% in 2012 (Fig. 10.3) (Center for Health Statistics and Information, 2013). However, as of 2013, non-public hospital beds made up only 15.6% of all beds, while outpatient and inpatients visits to private hospitals were 22.3% and 12%, respectively of total visits (State Council, 2014).

Fig. 10.3 Number of public and private hospitals by ownership, 2005–2012

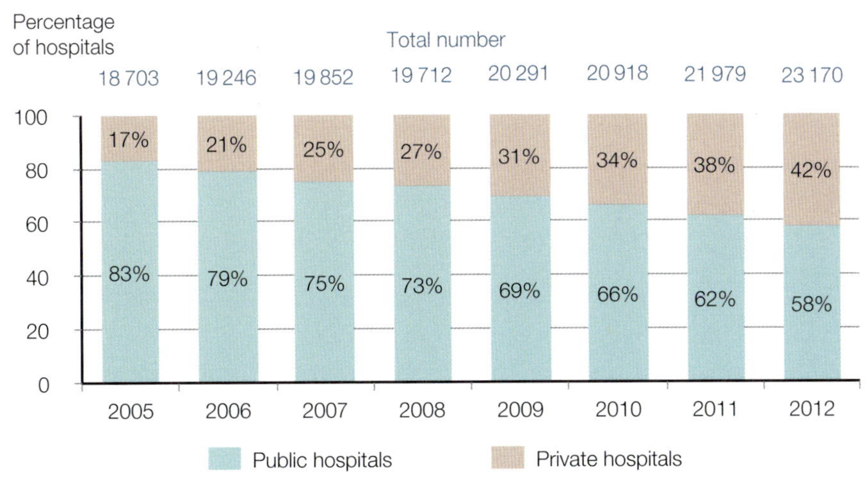

Source: Center for Health Statistics and Information, 2013.

Key challenges driving low utilization include low patient recognition, lack of qualified physicians, low public insurance coverage and historically weaker political support (Roland Berger, 2014). To this end, several favourable policies have been released that aim to increase the role of private hospitals in health service provision (Roland Berger, 2014):

- taxation: profit-making hospitals became exempt from corporate taxes in 2009;
- land and construction: qualified private hospitals are eligible for favourable land acquisition and construction policies;
- hospital rating: private hospitals are allowed to participate in hospital ratings alongside public hospitals;
- academics and R&D: private hospitals are encouraged to participate as teaching hospitals and the government also offers R&D support for building certain specializations seen as critical;

- professional qualifications: equal treatment of professional qualification and training for public and private hospitals; and
- capital type: diversified capital is encouraged in the structuring of private hospitals and there is no preference for domestic public, domestic private or foreign capital.

The government has also taken steps to explicitly limit the growth and role of public hospitals. In 2013, the NHFPC released "Several Opinions on Accelerating the Development of Medical Institutions Established by Social Capital", which actively sought to strip public hospitals of their dominance (NHFPC, 2013c). Policies regarding the flow of human resources between public and non-public hospitals, pricing of health services in non-public hospitals and insurance coverage for non-public hospitals have all facilitated the development of private hospitals.

In 2013, the NHFPC released the policy draft "Opinions on Multi-site Physician Practice", which outlined the conditions and limitations to multisite practice (NHFPC, 2014c). Traditionally, Chinese physicians have only been allowed to work at one medical facility. In this new guidance, physicians with more than five years of experience will be allowed to apply to work in more than one setting, although there are explicit stipulations to the amount of time that can be spent in non-public institutions. Lessons from abroad potentially point to an adverse effect on the quantity of care in the public sector when physicians are allowed to engage in dual practice. In the United Kingdom, the 25% of specialists who performed the most private work, largely financed by private health insurance and direct payments, carried out less NHS work than their colleagues (Audit Commission, 1995).

Prices in non-public hospitals are also subject to market forces, rather than being determined by the government as in public hospitals. Using market competition to regulate non-public hospital prices was first expressed in the 2013 NHFPC policy "Several Opinions on Accelerating the Development of Medical Institutions Established by Social Capital" (NHFPC, 2013c). This was later confirmed and expanded in greater detail by the "Notice Regarding the Issue of Using Market Regulation to Adjust Prices for Non-public Hospitals", jointly released by the NDRC, the NHFPC and the Ministry of Human Resources and Social Security in 2014. Specifically, the document stipulates "[non-public] medical institutions should price reasonably in accordance with the principles of fairness, good legal standing and good faith and maintain a relatively stable price level during a given period". In terms of insurance coverage, qualifying entities are allowed to deliver reimbursed care under the NCMS, UEBMI and URBMI schemes, private health insurance plans, workplace injury insurance and maternity insurance. Strategic purchasing is carried out via negotiations between the purchaser and the non-public provider to determine payment methods, tariffs and specifically to "increase the efficiency of funds".

The government has also sought to encourage foreign ownership of hospitals. The 70% maximum ownership constraint for foreign companies investing in private health care institutions was lifted in 2012 and led to a surge of health care-related public share activity. In total, RMB 3.2 billion was raised between May 2013 and August 2014, a huge increase compared with the RMB 0.4 billion raised through all of 2012 (Harrison & Yao, 2014). Investors preferred specialty hospitals covering such areas as plastic surgery, obstetrics/gynaecology and orthopaedics. Specialty hospitals, whose clinical capabilities are less comprehensive, do not require the large-scale investment general hospitals do. Second, many of the service items specialty hospitals offer are not reimbursable and, therefore, require more of the customized, high-margin offerings, with which public hospitals cannot compete (Roland Berger, 2014).

In spite of these favourable policies, private hospitals face significant challenges in assuming an expanded role as envisioned by the central government. Public hospital administrators are reluctant to share their best doctors, let alone see them leave permanently for private practice. Private providers have to pay a premium to bring in well-known clinicians, lure doctors from abroad or settle for younger doctors seeking a career boost (Harney, 2014)

10.10 Conclusions

Public hospital reform is one of the most challenging of all the health care reforms, given the central role hospitals play in the provision of care. On a broader health system level, China is probably too reliant on its hospitals and has too weak a primary care system. Addressing the entrenched incentive to overprescribe from the 15% mark-up policy is the main challenge hospital reformers face. While the government has made the removal of the link between drug sales and hospital revenues a priority, actually implementing this has proved very challenging. There has been disagreement across national ministries about how much of the revenue loss should be made up by government subsidies, and as a result the specifics of implementation have often been decided at a local level.

There have been several rounds of urban hospital reform, but their effects have been unclear because of a lack of strong evaluation data. County hospitals have implemented ZMU more broadly and have experienced some success in lowering drug revenues. However, funding shortfalls have been created from insufficient government subsidies and increases to medical service fees. Addressing shortfalls in direct funding for hospital operations and low physician salaries will be essential in creating a sustainable health care system. As the State Council is calling for universal adoption of ZMU in all urban hospitals by 2017 and significantly lower caps on total drug revenue and OOP spending, making up revenue gaps will become all the more pressing.

The central government has also recently been making a concerted effort to promote private hospitals. Various policies, such as favourable tax laws, allowing doctors to work in both public and private hospitals and lifting limits on foreign investment, have all been enacted in order to achieve the goal of 20% of care being provided at private hospitals by 2015. China must take steps to ensure that its private hospitals do not lead to a two-tiered system and that they actually do promote efficiency.

11. Primary care and pharmaceutical policy

KEY MESSAGES

- A strong primary care system can lead to better access, higher quality care, increased preventive activities and more efficient use of resources, particularly in China's specialist-driven system.
- The number of visits to primary care facilities has been increasing, but as a percentage of total health care visits is actually stagnating or decreasing.
- More should be done to promote the use of primary care, particularly in the face of rising rates of chronic diseases.
- The EDL and ZMU were introduced at the primary care level in order to decrease costs and encourage rational prescribing.
- There is evidence of reduced prices and more rational prescribing at the primary care level, although there is significant variation in effect sizes and it is unclear if price reductions persist.
- In order to make up for lost revenue from institution of ZMU, it is essential that the government increase subsidies to primary care facilities. These subsidies should ideally be linked to some measure of quality-related outcomes. Otherwise, unintended consequences such as unnecessary increased service provision may result.

11.1 An overview of primary care in China

Primary care is an essential part of any health care system. A strong primary care system can lead to greater access, higher quality care, an emphasis on prevention and more efficient use of health care resources (Starfield, Shi & Macinko, 2005). These are particularly salient in the Chinese context with its significant access inequalities, a rising burden of NCDs and increasing health care costs. China has made the development of a strong primary care system one of the five pillars of the 2009 health care reforms. Policy-makers envisioned a health care system anchored by CHCs in urban areas and THCs in rural areas, staffed by well-trained primary care staff who could serve as gatekeepers to higher levels of care (Liu et al., 2011). Unfortunately, China's current primary care system is very weak. People generally trust specialists and hospital care more than primary care, which tends to be staffed with relatively less educated workers and is underresourced.

Pharmaceutical and primary care policy are closely linked in China. The EDL was initially targeted at primary care to ensure that a package of essential medications was available at the most basic facilities at affordable prices. Primary care facilities were meant to mostly stock EDL medications to rein in the significant irrational prescribing at the primary care level. EDL use was initiated in tandem with the ZMU policy to decrease costs and to further deter irrational prescribing by removing the link between prescribing and revenue generation.

Before delving more deeply into the linkages between pharmaceuticals and primary care, it is important to understand the state of primary care in China. During the Mao era, China was a predominantly agrarian society. Health care was administered through the communes people lived and worked on through the Cooperative Medical Scheme. Barefoot doctors were the primary care providers and formed the backbone of the health care system (Blumenthal & Hsiao, 2005). These workers were well regarded internationally and effective at delivering care for rural populations at low cost with a focus on public health interventions (Zhang & Unschuld, 2008). This fairly robust primary care system collapsed with China's market liberalization reforms as public funding evaporated. Over the next two decades, primary care languished. The number of practitioners decreased as wages and prestige were poor, training opportunities were minimal and public trust in primary care decreased. Faced with rising health care costs and an increasing burden of chronic disease, interest in primary care began to grow. In 1997, the central government proposed piloting CHCs to provide care for its residents. In 2006, the State Council proposed using community health services as the anchor for the health care system, a sentiment enshrined in the 2009 reforms (Bhattacharyya et al., 2011).

In spite of this renewed leadership, there are significant challenges in building a strong primary care system. Decades of neglect have eroded public trust to the point where many seek care for simple ailments like a cold or hypertension at a tertiary hospital. Addressing the weakness of the primary care sector and at the same time reducing overreliance on hospitals is essential for efficient resource allocation in the health care system. There is significant overcrowding in China's urban hospitals, with doctors anecdotally seeing upwards of 60 patients a day (Ma & Adams, 2013). This limits the time available for effective diagnosis and management for each patient, with a focus instead on prescription writing and renewal.

There is a shortage of well-trained primary care providers, particularly in the rural and western regions of China (Liu et al., 2011). To address this personnel shortage, six ministries issued a joint plan in 2010 for capacity development and training (Dai et al., 2013) with the goal of training 300 000 family doctors by 2020 (Liu et al., 2011). China has also embarked on a significant infrastructure building programme: in 2012, the former health minister Chen Zhu claimed that the government had rebuilt a significant number of China's 2200 county hospitals and 33 000 urban and rural primary care facilities (Chen, 2012). In the latest urban hospital reform plan, the government has called for the creation of a "multilevel diagnosis and treatment service system", in which primary care facilities provide initial diagnostic and treatment services, with referrals to hospitals as necessary. The government hopes that 20% of public hospital visits will be through primary care referrals by the end of 2015 (State Council, 2015a).

11.2 Utilization of primary care

There were 8182 CHCs, 13 079 community nursing stations (these are satellite clinics of CHCs), and 37 097 THCs in 2011. In 2005, there were only 1382 CHCs, indicating a steady increase in the number of urban primary care facilities. However, there were 40 907 rural THCs in 2005, indicating that the number of THCs has been gradually decreasing (Fig. 11.1) (Center for Health Statistics and Information, 2014).

Fig. 11.1 Number of CHCs, THCs and community nursing stations, 2005–2013

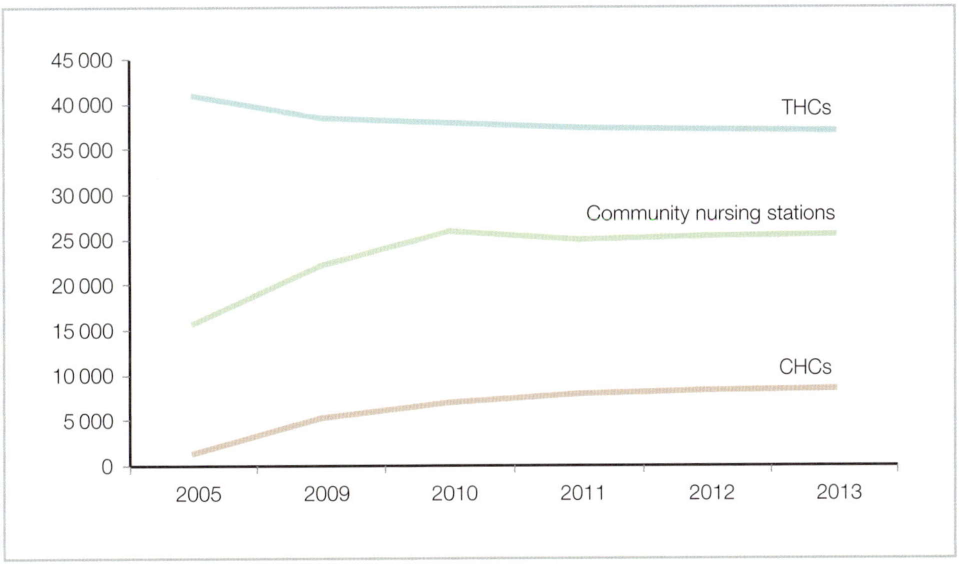

Source: Center for Health Statistics and Information, 2014.

There was a total of 4.324 billion visits to all primary care facilities in 2013, up from 2.594 billion in 2005 (Center for Health Statistics and Information, 2014). However, primary care visits as a percentage of all visits is actually declining. Primary care visits made up 63.3% of all visits in 2005 but only 59.1% by 2011 (Fig. 11.2) (Center for Health Statistics and Information, 2014). From these data, it would appear that patients were not switching from hospitals to primary care centres following the first few years of the reform.

In 2012, there were 109 794 general practitioners, including both physicians and physician assistants (Center for Health Statistics and Information, 2014). However, this figure masks a huge degree of heterogeneity in their training level.

Fig. 11.2 Visits to hospitals and primary care centres, 2005–2013

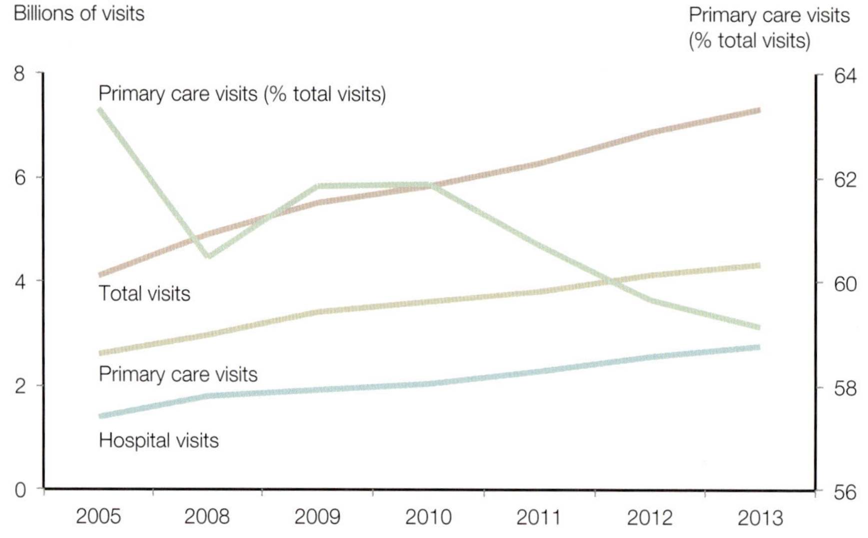

Source: Center for Health Statistics and Information, 2013.

11.3 Implementation of EDL and ZMU, government subsidies and unintended consequences

Pharmaceutical policies targeted at primary care can be broadly seen as serving three purposes: to ensure there is a quality supply of essential medications for patients, to improve affordability and to decrease the amount of irrational prescribing. When the EDL was first introduced, the government planned to implement it at 30% of primary care facilities by 2009 and 100% of facilities by 2012 (Guan et al., 2011). Primary care facilities were also seen as a springboard from which to expand the use of the EDL into higher-tier health care facilities. As of 2013, 98.8% of government-run primary care facilities had implemented the ZMU policy with EDL medications, suggesting the government did achieve a widespread rollout of the EDL (Hu, 2013).

Primary care facilities have traditionally generated a majority of their revenue from drug sales: THCs made 60.4% of outpatient revenues and 52.9% of inpatient revenues this way in 2010 (Zhang X et al., 2014). Implementation of ZMU would mean significant revenue loss through drug sales. To compensate for this loss in revenue, 90.2% of primary care facilities received government financial subsidies (Hu, 2013). A survey of 20 to 24 primary care facilities in each of six provinces demonstrated that the proportion of funding from the government increased significantly from 29.86% in 2010 to 38.84% in 2011. However, there was significant variation in funding across the six provinces, ranging from a low of 32.15% to a high of 53.40% in 2011 (Table 11.1) (Zhang X et al., 2013). There was also significant variation across individual facilities, with some receiving no funding and others receiving over RMB 13 million. Village clinics (one level down from THCs) have been particularly affected by ZMU, with a vast majority reporting a decline in income following implementation (Sun et al., 2014). Regional variation was also exacerbated through provinces making amendments to the initial 2009 iteration of the EDL; richer provinces could afford to add hundreds of items while a few poor ones added none. The expanded 2012 EDL was released with the stipulation that provinces would only be allowed to make minor adjustments (IMS Health, 2013b). These significant differences highlight the regional inequality endemic to China's health care system.

Table 11.1 Government financing for primary health care facilities in six provinces, 2010–2011

Province	Mean (minimum–maximum) (RMB thousands)	Government financing (% of total)	PMean (minimum–maximum) (RMB thousands)	Government financing (% of total)
Hubei	1 244 (30–5 160)	33.27	1 747 (130–7 830)	43.23
Lianoing	613 (0–4 139)	27.19	1 139 (50–6 400)	40.32
Shandong	852 (0–3 380)	19.36	1 806 (410–5 290)	35.36
Shanxi	409 (20–1 920)	34.00	549 (30–2 740)	35.23
Shaanxi	1 102 (100–2 372)	48.80	1 225 (90–2 750)	53.40
Sichuan	1 034 (37–12 715)	29.50	1 239 (0–13 080)	32.15
Average	**881**	**29.86**	**1 300**	**38.84**

Source: Zhang X et al., 2013.

Implementation of ZMU with its associated revenue losses have led to unintended consequences as physicians seek to make up for revenue through other means. A qualitative study of rural physicians working in six provinces revealed large changes in doctor income structure following ZMU, with decreased drug revenue and increased reliance on government salaries and subsidies (Zhang S et al., 2015). Survey results indicate that compensation levels were often lower and that many doctors continued to sell drugs with a mark-up in secret to compensate for this. Another study of THCs found a significant shift towards medical services following ZMU implementation. Among those THCs with greater baseline reliance on drug revenues, the share of drug revenue declined by 43% but the number of inpatients treated increased by 127%, leading to an overall small increase in total revenue (Yi et al., 2015). As revenue from drug sales decreases, it would be prudent to monitor for these unintended consequences and attempt to channel funding for primary care facilities and physicians towards activities that improve care.

11.4 Review of effects of EDL and ZMU on prescribing and drug costs

Many studies have assessed the impact of EDL and ZMU as well as other policy changes at the primary care level. Key outcomes of these studies have been rates of irrational prescribing, costs faced by patients and patient satisfaction. Table 11.2 summarizes the studies looking at the effect of the EDL and ZMU policies on cost and prescribing.

Table 11.2 Summary of studies studying effect of EDL/ZMU on primary care facilities

Study	Study scope	Cost outcomes	Irrational prescribing outcomes
Yao et al., 2015	CHCs and THCs in a central China province	Average cost per prescription decreased from RMB 42 to RMB 28 in CHCs and RMB 43 to RMB 33 in THCs	Negligible changes in the rates of antibiotic, steroid and injection prescribing
Song et al., 2014a	THCs in Shandong, Zhejiang, Anhui and Ningxia provinces from 2009 to 2011 (pre–post)	Median decrease of 34.4% in drug prices in 2010 compared with 2009; however, more expensive drugs were prescribed more often post-EDL	Not assessed

Table 11.2 Summary of studies studying effect of EDL/ZMU on primary care facilities (continued)

Study	Study scope	Cost outcomes	Irrational prescribing outcomes
Song et al., 2014b	THCs in Shandong, Zhejiang, Anhui and Ningxia provinces from 2009 to 2010 (pre–post)	Cost per prescription increased from RMB25.77 to RMB27.09	Percentage of prescriptions for antibiotics fell from 60.26% to 58.48%; the percentage of treatments with injections fell from 42.93% to 40.31%
Zhang X et al., 2014	196 THCs in Chongqing, Henan and Jiangsu from 2009 to 2010 (pre–post)	Decline in inpatient drug expenditure by 26% and total expenditure by 10%; no change in outpatient expenditure	Not assessed
Chen et al., 2014	83 CHCs and THCs around the country from 2007 to 2010 (difference-in-difference analysis)	In urban CHCs, the average expenditure for EDL group fell from RMB92.37 to RMB66.07 compared with RMB69.36 to RMB58.22 for non-EDL group. In rural CHCs, EDL group fell from RMB33.72 to RMB31.53 compared with an increase from RMB29.27 to RMB33.52 for the non-EDL group	Decreasing use of injections for hypertension but still increasing use of antibiotics; increase in antibiotics less in EDL arm than non-EDL arm
Tang et al., 2013	126 primary care facilities in six provinces (propensity score matching)	Not assessed	In facilities with higher subsidies, the likelihood of receiving an injection was 33.79%, compared with 42.12% in facilities with lower subsidies

Table 11.2 Summary of studies studying effect of EDL/ZMU on primary care facilities (continued)

Study	Study scope	Cost outcomes	Irrational prescribing outcomes
Yang et al., 2012	18 primary care facilities in Hubei province (with parallel controls)	Average expenditure per prescription decreased from RMB 44.67 to RMB 26.67	No significant reduction antibiotic or injection use
Cheng et al., 2012	351 Beijing CHCs from 2006 to 2009	Initial decrease in cost per visit of 18.7% from 2006 to 2007 in the most subsidized CHCs; however, by 2009, prices had increased from baseline by 6.3%; larger price increases in CHCs receiving less government subsidy	Not assessed
Xiang et al., 2012	120 primary care facilities in Liaoning, Shandong, Hubei, Shanxi, Sichuan and Shaanxi provinces from 2010 to 2011	Not assessed	Average percentage of prescriptions with an injection decreased from 38.91% to 36.82%

Irrational prescribing

An early study assessing the effects of the EDL on irrational prescribing in primary care looked at the misuse of injections at 120 primary care facilities in six provinces (Xiang et al., 2012). Questionnaires sent to these facilities asked about changes in the percentage of prescriptions with injections between 2010 and 2011. The authors reported a small but statistically significant decline from 38.91% to 36.82%. Nevertheless, injection use was still far in excess of WHO guidelines, which recommend rates of 13–25%. Government subsidy of primary care facilities – an important counterpart to the ZMU policy – was shown to reduce the number of prescriptions for injections (Tang et al., 2013). The rate of prescriptions in "high-subsidy" facilities was 33.79% compared with 42.12% in "low-subsidy" facilities. Some studies have shown less promising results: A study of rural and urban primary care facilities in Hubei Province demonstrated that while uptake of EDL medications was quite high at 95% there was no reduction in irrational prescribing, with

68% of all prescriptions still containing an antibiotic (Yang et al., 2012). One of the more recent studies demonstrated only a small reduction in antibiotic prescribing, from 60.26% to 58.48% of all prescriptions, but larger reductions in injections and adrenal corticosteroids, from 40.31% to 11.16% (Song et al., 2014b). Another study demonstrated negligible changes in the prescribing of antibiotics, steroids and injections in CHCs and THCs (Yao et al., 2015).

Medication costs

The linkages between ZMU, government subsidies and drug costs were explored in a study of Beijing CHCs (Cheng et al., 2012). In wealthier areas of Beijing, which received subsidies covering all personnel and clinic costs, EDL drug costs decreased by 18.7% following implementation; this compares with only 1.9% in poorer areas where subsidies covered only staff and not clinic costs. This study showed that in later years prices of EDL medications actually rebounded to higher than baseline levels. A later study of primary care facilities in four provinces demonstrated a significant average decrease in EDL prices of 34.4% (Song et al., 2014a). Interestingly, there was also an increase in prescribing of more expensive drugs, perhaps to compensate for overall price decreases. One study found there was a decline in inpatient, but not outpatient, drug expenditure (Zhang X et al., 2014). Another study with a control non-EDL arm found that there were greater decreases in patient drug expenses in both urban and rural primary care facilities that implemented EDL versus those that did not (Chen et al., 2014). Yet another study found a decrease in average cost per prescription in both CHCs and THCs, although declines were larger in urban areas (Yao et al., 2015).

Patient satisfaction

A 2011 study of Shanghai CHCs looked at patient satisfaction across a number of domains following the 2009 reforms (Li et al., 2012). In terms of medication access, half of patients believed that access had decreased or not changed while only a third felt that it had improved. Indeed, the overall satisfaction score with the essential medication system was lower than that for other domains such as clinical services. These results are particularly problematic as Shanghai has one of the most advanced and well-funded primary care systems in China.

11.5 Conclusions

Recognizing the important role primary care has to play within a health care system, China has made strengthening its primary care system one of the priorities of the health care reforms. Health care provision in China is dominated by hospitals, and preliminary data following the reforms suggest that there has not been a shift away from hospitals to primary care. Major barriers include lack of well-trained personnel and a lack of public trust with primary care in general. A strong primary system will be essential in helping China to deal with its burden of NCDs, as primary care providers are capable of providing high-quality, accessible care in a cost-effective manner.

Primary care has been the testing ground for many key pharmaceutical policies such as the EDL and the ZMU policy. Such policies are seen as essential in promoting basic medications that are affordable and accessible while reducing irrational prescribing. So far, it seems these policies have been somewhat successful in decreasing the prices of medications; equivocal in terms of their effects on irrational prescribing, with only small decreases in antibiotic and injection use; and not very successful at actually improving patient satisfaction and patients' perceptions of affordability.

As government seeks to rationalize the pharmaceutical environment through ZMU, it is important to consider the financial situation faced by primary care facilities. Income lost from ZMU must be made up through government subsidies or alternative funding mechanisms in order for reforms to be sustainable and to promote and grow primary care. Many facilities appear to have faced revenue shortfalls and there has been significant inequality in the extent to which lost drug revenues are supplemented by the relevant governments. There has been some evidence of unintended increases in the number of medical encounters to make up for lost revenue. Ideally funding could be linked to value (e.g. effective prescribing or effective medical services). Given the benefits that a strong primary care system can bring, the government would do well to continue to support continued development of primary care through pharmaceutical policies.

12. Pharmacies and pharmacists

KEY MESSAGES

- The pharmacy sector is growing rapidly, driven by policies to encourage more drug sales outside of hospitals, increasing demand for health care and better insurance coverage.
- As reforms to remove the link between drug sales and hospital revenues progress, the role of community pharmacies and drugstores is set to expand. However, regulation will be necessary to ensure hospitals do not enter profit-sharing agreements with pharmacies.
- Pharmacists can play an important role in both the community and hospitals. They can provide patient education, engage in health-promotion activities and encourage rational prescribing and the use of safe and cost-effective medications.
- There are a number of barriers to increasing the number of pharmacies and pharmacists. These include a relatively limited number of training programmes, a workforce skewed towards working for drug manufacturers rather than providing clinical care and a lack of awareness about the role and capabilities of pharmacists.
- Online pharmacies will experience rapid growth following a relaxation of CFDA regulations. Since 2012, sales have increased ten-fold and e-retailing will compete with physical stores in the growing pharmacy market.

12.1 Trends in retail pharmacy revenues in China

While pharmaceutical sales have traditionally been dominated by hospitals, China's retail pharmacy sector is growing rapidly. Retail pharmacies offer another avenue by which drug sales can be separated from hospitals and they can potentially be more convenient and accessible for patients. Average sales growth has been 19.1% since 2010 and total revenues are forecasted to reach slightly over RMB 1 trillion by 2020 (Fig. 12.1) (IBISWorld, 2015b). Only about 50% of revenue is derived from the sale of prescription medications, with the other half coming from OTC medications and other personal products (IBISWorld, 2015b). As with overall pharmaceutical spending, growth in retail pharmacy revenues is projected to decline over the next several years.

Fig. 12.1 Annual revenues and year-on-year growth of retail pharmacies, 2006–2014 and projections to 2020

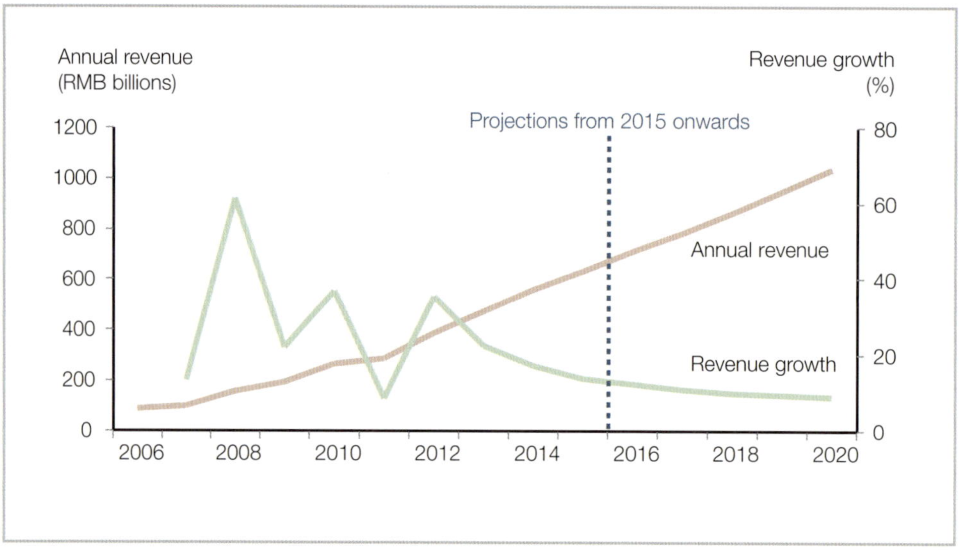

Source: IBISWorld, 2015b.

Growth in the pharmacy industry is being driven by a number of factors: rising disposable incomes, better insurance coverage, high drug prices in hospitals, consumers' ability to self-medicate, increasing foreign investment after China's accession to the World Trade Organization in 2001 and the government's support for the development of chain drug-retailing enterprises (IBISWorld, 2015b). In spite of these growth forecasts, profits are expected to account for only 5.2% of industry revenue in 2015 (IBISWorld, 2015b). This reflects a high degree of competition between pharmacies as they seek to differentiate themselves by the services they provide. As with China's drug-manufacturing industry, the retail pharmacy sector is highly fragmented. The top 100 chains had only about 20% of total market share by revenue in 2015 (IBISWorld, 2015b).

In order to earn more profits, many companies have emphasized their non-pharmaceutical offerings, particularly cosmetics (IBISWorld, 2015b). Recent examples of success in this area include Taiwan's Cosmed; Hong Kong's two chains, Watsons and Mannings; and Hongzhou Wulin Drugstore. China's lengthy pharmaceutical supply chains also means that various distributors capture parts of the margin. As urban competition increases, more pharmacies will expand to rural areas, where they can hopefully improve access to drugs. Chain drug retailers will also expand in order to obtain economies of scale with associated cost savings.

12.2 Pharmacies and removing the linkage of drug sales with hospitals

Currently, over 70% of drugs are sold through hospitals, but reforms are being introduced that will force hospitals to focus on providing medical services rather than selling drugs (State Council, 2015d). Hospitals currently derive around 40% of their revenues from drug sales. With the 2015 State Council work plan calling for drug sales to account for a maximum of 30% of hospital revenues, the capacity for pharmacies to expand will be greatly enhanced. A government official from Guangdong Province predicted that eventually pharmacies will become a cost rather than a profit centre for hospitals as they will no longer be generating revenues (Woodhead, 2014). This should help to remove hospital incentives to overprescribe in order to increase profits, one of the key themes of the health reforms.

Regulation will still be needed to ensure that hospitals do not simply create profit-sharing arrangements with these detached pharmacies and thus restore the incentive for overprescription. These pharmacies could be extremely lucrative for pharmaceutical companies. Kangmei Pharmaceutical has already signed contracts to manage the pharmacies and supply all pharmaceuticals within hospitals in areas such as Liaoning and Guangdong (Yang, 2014).

12.3 Retail pharmacies in the community

Community pharmacies have convenient locations, easy accessibility and play a critical role in ensuring access to health services. Their responsibilities have gradually been increasing from medication dispensing to include the provision of pharmaceutical services (Fang et al., 2013). These services include tasks such as patient education and monitoring medication profiles. Health care reforms have also emphasized the responsibility of pharmacists to encourage the use of low-cost medications and promote the rational use of medications. It is important to keep in mind that pharmacists must be compensated appropriately in order to encourage them to engage in these sorts of counselling activities. This requires a careful balance in dispensing fees and counselling fees.

According to the "12th Five Year Plan on Drug Safety and Standards" released by the State Council in 2012, newly opened community pharmacies must be staffed by licensed pharmacists during business hours to ensure the quality of medications and services (State Council, 2012a). Furthermore, all community pharmacies should be owned by licensed pharmacists by the end of 2015. These ambitious targets require an expanded pharmacy workforce. Unfortunately, in general, there is a relative shortage of both pharmacies and pharmacists. For example, in China there were 377 000 hospital pharmacists in 2012, or an average of 279 per million people – far lower than the OECD average of 890 per million (Center for Health Statistics and Information, 2013). The pharmacy workforce is also skewed towards manufacturing and hospitals rather than the community: as of 2006, 80% of pharmacists worked in manufacturing and in hospitals while less than 10% worked in the community (Philipsen, 2013).

A number of factors other than personnel shortages present barriers to the effective delivery of community pharmacy services (Fang et al., 2011). A survey of community pharmacists in Shaanxi Province highlighted a number of challenges to patient-oriented pharmacy service provision, including insufficient time to spend with patients, a lack of proper skills and training, limited economic incentives and lack of support from other health care workers.

The State Council is facilitating the expansion of chain pharmacies, which have been successful at providing medicines and quality service to patients (*PR Newswire*, 2015). New regulations allow for more rapid expansion of chains in the form of faster approvals for newly acquired storefronts. These regulations are aimed at increasing the market concentration of companies able to adhere to high standards of quality.

12.4 Broadening use of clinical pharmacy services in hospitals

Within the hospital setting, pharmacists can play an important role in rational prescribing and the use of cost-effective therapies. Indeed, there is evidence that the use of pharmacist services can decrease the prescribing of unnecessary antibiotics and cut costs in a hospital setting (Zhang H-X et al., 2014). A similar study also demonstrated that involving pharmacists decreased the cost and duration of inpatient admissions for respiratory tract infections (Shen et al., 2011a). A literature review found pharmacist services had a positive effect on rational prescribing and patient care (Penm et al., 2013). Three crucial themes govern the further adoption of pharmacist services within hospitals (Penm et al., 2014):

External and systemic factors. Government and hospital administrative support is essential for the implementation of pharmacist services. Physicians may be writing prescriptions for medicolegal reasons rather than for rational clinical use and they should be encouraged to pay more heed to pharmacists. Adoption of standardized clinical pathways can facilitate the role of pharmacists in promoting rational medication use.

Resources for clinical pharmacy. There is a shortage of pharmacists throughout China. Increasing pharmacy education should help to increase the number and quality of pharmacists who are able to work in hospitals.

Awareness of clinical pharmacists. Patients are often unaware of the concept of clinical pharmacy and do not understand the role of clinical pharmacists. This hinders service utilization.

Potential strategies for aiding the implementation of clinical pharmacy services within hospitals include (Penm et al., 2014):

- expanding the role of pharmacists in promoting medication safety;
- expanding the role of pharmacists in patient education;
- engaging in more medical research; and

- increasing the use of pharmacy technicians and dispensing machines so that pharmacists can focus on more clinically oriented tasks.

Survey data suggest that physicians are quite supportive of an increased role for pharmacists in the hospital setting particularly when it comes to providing patient-oriented services or in supporting physician decision-making (Li et al., 2014).

12.5 Pharmacy education and licensing in China

In order to increase the role of pharmacists in the community and in hospitals, more well-trained pharmacists are needed. Clinical pharmacy programmes are relatively new to China; they were first established in 1989 but developed more fully after 2006 (Hu et al., 2014). In 2012, there were 30 pharmacy colleges with clinical pharmacy undergraduate programmes, more than 40 colleges offering master's programmes and five universities offering doctorate programmes. However, pharmacy programmes in China are pharmacologically oriented rather than patient oriented, with an emphasis on basic science rather than on patient and clinical interaction (Yi et al., 2014). In order to develop well-trained clinical pharmacists, programmes must move towards teaching both aspects of pharmacy.

There are a few major barriers facing undergraduate clinical pharmacy education in China (Hu et al., 2014). First, the structure and content of the clinical pharmacy curriculum needs to be improved to make it more practical and systematic. Second, practical elements of clinical pharmacy programmes need to be improved – students lack the chance to consolidate theoretical knowledge and find it hard to adjust when they enter practice. Lastly, curricular development efforts need input from practising pharmacists in the community and in hospitals, as these are the people who are most aware of the demands put on them in the working world. Several measures are being taken to improve clinical pharmacy education (Hu et al., 2014). There is support for the establishment of more clinical pharmacy programmes and ongoing efforts to establish accreditation standards and guidelines for programmes across the country. More colleges are recognizing these curricular challenges and are engaging in pilot reforms. Cooperation between pharmacy programmes and hospitals will further improve the quality of education. Ideally more faculty members will have a clinical pharmacy background, and hospital pharmacists will be involved in teaching college courses.

In China, licensed pharmacists are those professionals who pass the annually held unified national examination and obtain the Licensed Pharmacist Certificate (Fudong & Boyang, 2011). They are responsible for the quality of drugs and uphold basic principles of safe and effective drug use. A second system also exists, under which a pharmacy worker is assigned a specialist title (such as chief pharmacist, associate chief pharmacist, pharmacist in-charge, pharmacist or assistant pharmacist), according to their educational background, work experience and professional skills. The majority of licensed pharmacists work for drug distributors and manufacturers, while the majority of specialist pharmacists work in medical institutions. In terms of geographical distribution, most registered licensed pharmacists are employed in the eastern and middle parts of China, while much fewer work in the western regions.

The educational and licensing landscape for pharmacists in China can be improved in a number of ways (Fudong & Boyang, 2011). First, more licensed pharmacists should be trained to meet rising demand in hospitals and in the community. In doing so, educational standards must be upheld (Box 12.1). Second, there should be a unified licensing system and standards for both licensed pharmacists (who tend to work in distributors and manufacturers) and for specialist pharmacists (who tend to work in medical facilities). Third, any unified licensing system should incorporate more clinical and patient-oriented elements rather than the current emphasis on drug pharmacology.

Box 12.1 Cheating on the pharmacy unified national examination

In the 2014 sitting of the pharmacy unified national examination in Xi'an, Shaanxi Province, 2440 students were caught cheating across seven test centres. Approximately 10% of all test-takers in the province were involved in the cheating. Those found cheating have been banned from taking the test for two years.

Currently Shaanxi has 4000 licensed pharmacists. National regulations stipulate that pharmacies and distributors must have at least one licensed pharmacist, but as there are 8500 such firms there simply are not enough pharmacists to go around. As a result, there is huge pressure to train more licensed pharmacists. However, the licensing process, which requires candidates to pass seven 150-minute examinations within a two-year window, is highly competitive. It is likely that the combination of increasing demand for pharmacists coupled with an extremely challenging examination contributed to the cheating (Christiansen, 2014; Press Trust of India, 2014).

12.6 Online pharmacies in China

For many years, the online sale of drugs has been highly regulated in China. Only a few pharmacy chains with store outlets could sell online to consumers and the large e-retailing giants such as Alibaba were only licensed to provide information on medications to patients. In spite of this, online pharmacies are undergoing a period of unprecedented growth in China. In 2014, online sales increased to an estimated RMB 3.9 billion, an almost ten-fold increase from 2011 sales (McTiernan, 2014b).

In May 2014, the CFDA released a draft update to pharmaceutical e-retailing guidelines that opened the door for online sales of prescription drugs and medical devices and eased licensing requirements for third-party platforms such as Alibaba. These new guidelines have the potential to usher in even more explosive growth in online drug sales in China.

Online pharmacies can make shopping for medications and price comparisons easier for the patient and should intensify competition among traditional pharmacy chains and hopefully drive down prices. The government also hopes that "consumer democracy", in which patients now have more choice in where to purchase their medications, will further their goals of limiting drug sales in hospitals.

The specifics around the new regulations remain nebulous. Currently sales are limited to an online-to-offline model, in which patients may buy online but must pick up their drugs at a physical store. There is also a requirement for online pharmacists to be available to answer patient questions. Both of these requirements will limit the growth of online sales but can be seen as important in ensuring drug quality and patient safety (Jourdan, 2015). Regulation will be particularly important as some evidence suggests that a large proportion of online retailers are not abiding by Chinese laws or regulations (Alliance for Safe Online Pharmacies, 2015).

12.7 Conclusions

Traditionally, retail pharmacies are a much weaker part of the health care sector compared with developed countries but they have experienced significant growth over recent years. The government is encouraging their development as entities independent from hospitals as another means through which drug sales can be unlinked from hospitals. Ambitious targets that will limit the revenue hospitals can derive from drug sales mean that pharmacies will have a promising growth avenue.

Community pharmacies can provide a more accessible location for patients to acquire their medications. Recent changes to CFDA guidelines will significantly promote the growth of online pharmacies. These e-retailers will compete with traditional stores and also contribute to increased access and affordability, but regulation for this nascent sector will be important to ensure quality. Competition between community pharmacies, hospitals and online pharmacies could help to decrease prices for patients. The use of clinical pharmacy services is also being encouraged throughout hospitals, where studies have demonstrated the ability of pharmacist interventions to decrease antibiotic use and lower overall health care costs.

Unfortunately, China faces a huge shortage in the number of trained and qualified pharmacists. Education programmes and licensing systems will need to be strengthened to meet increasing demand. A recent cheating scandal on the national pharmacy licensing examination demonstrates that in the face of increased pressure to train more pharmacists quality and integrity must be maintained.

13. Traditional Chinese medicine

KEY MESSAGES

- TCM has been used in China for thousands of years. In recent decades, attempts have been made at modernizing its use but there are still huge gaps in our understanding of these drugs.
- A majority of the population has used TCM, and TCMs account for about 30% of TPE. China's TCM hospitals tend to offer western services and western hospitals also offer TCM services.
- As with western medicines, TCM is regulated by the CFDA. The regulation of TCM is challenging because of product heterogeneity and varied manufacturing processes.
- There are significant concerns about TCM safety and quality. The less standardized nature of TCM preparations and the multitude of points at which contamination can occur contribute to this.
- Drug interactions are an area of potential danger, particularly as the mechanisms of action of many TCMs are not well elucidated and interactions with other TCMs and western medications are difficult to predict.
- The government is keen to promote the export of TCM, and consumers in other countries are quite receptive. As the export market grows, other jurisdictions have sought to regulate TCMs in order to protect consumers but they face many of the same challenges as Chinese authorities.

13.1 Introduction to TCM

TCM is a holistic system for diagnosis, prevention and treatment that has existed for thousands of years. The underlying theory of disease underlying TCM is completely different from that of western medicine. From a treatment perspective, TCM incorporates acupuncture and the use of herbal preparations. This chapter will focus on the use of herbal preparations: the "pharmaceutical" side of TCM. While there is a vast theoretical gap between TCM and western medicine, some of its treatment modalities have demonstrated efficacy. For example, a recent meta-analysis of trials showed that real acupuncture was more effective than sham acupuncture in the treatment of chronic pain (Vickers et al., 2012). Many different western medications also have their basis in TCMs: in 2015, the Nobel Prize for Medicine was awarded to Youyou Tu for the discovery of a common malaria treatment, artemisinin, which was derived from the traditionally used herb *Artemisia annua* (Miller & Su, 2011).

Although the origins of TCM theory can be traced back to *Huangdi's Internal Classic* from around 475–211 BC, it is only recently that attempts have been made to modernize its practice (Cheung, 2011). This process started in the 1950s, when China began establishing a network of TCM universities, hospitals and research institutions. Between 1954 and 1960, China's ten most prestigious TCM universities and its national TCM academy were established. Meanwhile, from 1949 to 1984, there was almost a 3000% increase in the number of beds in TCM hospitals (Xu et al., 2013). TCM was used extensively by China's barefoot doctors during this time. In 1985, the State Administration of Chinese Medicine was established as a national coordinating body for TCM-related issues. From the 1980s onwards, there has been increasing interest in integrating TCM with western medicine. There has also been significant international interest in TCM. Western nations have been keen to import TCMs as well as to initiate research programmes into their effectiveness.

In spite of the many TCM success stories and attempts at modernization, the evidence base for the majority of TCM preparations is limited or non-existent. It is not clear what percentage of TCM remedies are effective. Guaranteeing quality, safety and standardization is very challenging, even more so than with western medications given that with the latter there is usually only one active ingredient per drug whereas an herbal preparation can contain numerous active compounds. Finally, there is a limited understanding of drug interactions between TCM and western medicines, which can lead to major safety concerns.

13.2 Use of TCM in China

Although the use of western medicines is increasing, TCM still plays an important role in China's health care and continues to receive strong government support. Within China's 12th Five Year Plan for the TCM industry, the government promised to increased coverage of TCM services, train more TCM practitioners, encourage the uptake of TCM by patients and continue to fund research and promote national and international collaborations in furthering the understanding of TCM (L.E.K., 2012). Approximately 60% of the population has consulted a TCM practitioner at least once (Cheung, 2011). In 2013, there were 810 million visits to TCM institutions, up from 476 million in 2008 (Center for Health Statistics and Information, 2014). There were close to 49 000 TCM treatment facilities in China in 2013, up from about 27 500 in 2008 (Center for Health Statistics and Information, 2014). Indeed, TCM-related services make up about 18% of total health care provision in China (Qiu, 2015). In practice, there is significant blurring of provision between TCM and western medical services. For example, the vast majority of western hospitals, up to 90%, have TCM departments; similarly, western medicine is commonly practised in TCM hospitals (Xu & Yang, 2009).

TCM drugs made up approximately 30% of TPE in 2012 (Niu, 2015) and they have a particularly high market share in the retail pharmacy setting. They made up 44% of total pharmacy drug sales: 32% for prescription TCM and 12% for OTC sales in 2013 (Niu, 2015). Between 2007 and 2012, multiple sources found that growth in TCM sales was between 20% and 25% (DBS Group Research, 2015; Euromonitor, 2014; Niu, 2015). However, by 2014, growth had decreased to about 12%, in line with a general decline in the rate of drug spending increases (Niu, 2015). Drugs for cardiovascular diseases are the top-selling prescription TCMs while those for respiratory diseases are the top-selling OTC TCMs, which reflects the perception that they are best suited for chronic diseases (Niu, 2015). The consumption of TCMs are generally higher in lower-tier health facilities and in rural areas.

From a reimbursement perspective, a large number of TCM preparations are covered under both the EDL (39%) and the NRDL (46%). Even though a substantial proportion of the two major reimbursement lists are made up of TCMs, there is a dearth of evidence guiding the selection of products for inclusion. In principle, products must demonstrate benefit in the management, prevention and control of disease, but in practice it appears that the government relies heavily on the opinions of expert TCM practitioners (Fang et al., 2013). A survey of 137 experts from 31 medical and research institutions involved in TCM highlighted that key factors in deciding upon reimbursement should be patient preference, evidence on long-term outcomes, comparative studies with western medicines and safety and side-effect profiles (Zhang F et al., 2013). Experts also felt that information on cost–effectiveness was crucial, although little currently exists.

While most Chinese have used TCM, surveys have demonstrated that western medicine is preferred. A 2003 survey revealed that 52% of patients preferred western medicine alone, 25% preferred integrated TCM/western treatment, 12% preferred TCM treatment alone, and the remainder preferred either TCM or western treatment based on the chronicity of their condition (Xu & Yang, 2009). These preferences are borne out by changes in the revenue streams of hospitals. A survey of 97 TCM hospitals from around China found that the percentage of revenues derived from offering western medicine increased from 44.3% to 47.4% between 1999 and 2004, while the revenues derived from TCM fell from 26.4% to 18.8% during the same period (Shen et al., 2011b). National statistics demonstrate a similar decline in TCM drug revenue as a percentage of total drug revenue among hospitals. Between 1999 and 2008, TCM drug revenue at TCM hospitals declined from 18.0% to 13.7% of total drug revenue (Shen et al., 2011b). TCM faces stiff competition from western medication for a number of reasons, including the broader scope of care offered by western medicine (e.g. laboratory testing and surgery), the delayed effects of TCM compared with western medicines and the superiority of western medicines in treating acute conditions.

13.3 Regulation of TCM

The regulation of TCM is more challenging as the products themselves are less standardized and their use is not as deeply grounded in the scientific literature (Zhang et al.,

2012). Herbal medicines can broadly be divided into three groups: raw herbal medicines, sliced herbal medicines and patent medicines. Sliced herbal medicines are those that have been processed past their raw forms while patent medicines are more standardized, rather than patented per se (Zhang et al., 2012).

The CFDA is responsible for registering new TCM drugs and in principle they are subject to similar technical evaluations as western medicines, including having data on effectiveness and safety. However, TCM preparations with a long history of use can be exempted from some of these requirements (Wu W-Y et al., 2014). Those seeking market authorizations for TCM preparations apply for one of nine categories (Table 13.1) (Wu W-Y et al., 2014).

Table 13.1 Registration categories for TCM drugs seeking market authorization

Category	Description	Notes
1	Active ingredients and their preparations extracted from plants, animals, minerals or other substances which have not been marketed in China	Drugs in this category include artemisinin for malaria and arsenic trioxide for the treatment of leukaemia
2	Newly discovered crude drugs and their preparations	Includes drugs not yet recognized as medicines of any national, provincial or autonomous region, or municipal jurisdiction; few TCMs are registered here
3	New substitutes of existing Chinese drugs	Involves replacing crude drugs in TCM preparations that are toxic or are in danger of extinction; few TCMs are registered here
4	New medicinal parts of existing crude drugs or their preparations	Requires using different parts of traditional TCM products (e.g. the rhizomes and rootlets of Panax notoginseng) in addition to the traditionally used roots; few TCMs are registered here
5	Active fractions and their preparations extracted from plants, animals, minerals or other substances that have not been marketed in China	The pharmacologically active components must make up more than 50% of extracts; although these are simpler than complex TCM preparations, these are still mixtures of chemicals, which may require multicomponent quality control and pharmacokinetic testing

Table 13.1 Registration categories for TCM drugs seeking market authorization (continued)

Category	Description	Notes
6	Preparations of TCM formulas and natural medicine formulas that have not been marketed in China	Some medicines under this category are considered safe and efficacious because of a long history of use and can bypass phase I and II clinical studies; other medicines under this category include mixtures of chemical medicines and have more strict testing requirements
7	Preparations with altered mode of drug delivery of marketed Chinese medicines and natural medicine products	Categories 7, 8 and 9 are for products that are already on the market but with a change in mode of administration (category 7), change in dosage (category 8) or no change at all (category 9)
8	Preparations with altered dosage form of drug delivery of marketed Chinese medicines and natural medicine products	
9	Generics	

Source: Wu W-Y et al., 2014.

Intellectual property protection for TCMs is conceptually challenging, as many recipes are public knowledge or recorded in books that have been passed down for thousands of years (Jiang, 2011). China started awarding patents for TCM drugs in the 1990s, although it is not entirely clear what governs which drugs are eligible for patent protection. Unfortunately, patents for new drugs can sometimes be obtained by very minor changes to a product or even to its packaging (Jiang, 2011).

As with western medicines, there is significant market fragmentation, with thousands of manufacturers of TCM products (Xu & Yang, 2009). This further contributes to challenges in quality control and the regulatory burden faced by the CFDA. The heterogeneous nature of many TCM preparations makes quality control more challenging than for western medications. As many products are plant based, even variation in growing conditions and climate can affect the final product. This is the case for both TCM injections as well as oral medications (Qiu, 2015). The government has introduced various mechanisms such as Good Agricultural Practice, Good Laboratory Practice and

GMP, but implementation is challenging. The standards for the ingredient mix in patent medicines and for the preparation processes involved in sliced herbal medicines are not clearly delineated. As a result, manufacturers can cut costs by using less effective components in their products (Xu & Yang, 2009).

13.4 Safety of TCM

There is a common misperception that because something is "herbal" or "natural" it is, therefore, safe. This is patently untrue. Like any medication, TCMs can have positive therapeutic effects but also can cause significant harm if used inappropriately. An example of this was the causal relationship found between aristolochic acid, a compound found in a TCM weight-loss remedy, and renal fibrosis and eventual renal cell carcinoma among Belgian women in the early 1990s (De Broe, 2012). TCM safety is a major concern among patients. A survey of hundreds of community pharmacies in Guangzhou and Shanghai, two of China's largest cities, assessed the key determinants in consumers' preferences for OTC TCM products (Ge, He & Hu, 2014). It found that medication safety was the most influential factor and that even drug side-effects were more important than drug price or brand.

Safety and quality problems can arise for many reasons for TCM. Broadly speaking, these can be summarized into drug-specific factors and clinical-use factors (Table 13.2) (Zhang et al., 2012). Conceptually, maintaining the safety of TCM is more difficult than for western medicines. TCM is less standardized (i.e. different growing, preparation, storage conditions); preparations often contain a mixture of active ingredients, and there is less evidence on safety, mechanism of action, pharmacokinetics and so on.

The possibility of drug interactions is particularly concerning because of the increased use of both western medicines and TCM as well as a lack of strong pharmacological understanding of many TCM products. There is an increasing number of databases that contain information on the active chemicals found within TCM preparations (Chan et al., 2010). However, predicting drug interactions remains quite challenging. Interactions can occur between a TCM preparation and other TCMs (herb–herb interactions) or between a TCM preparation and western drugs (herb–drug interactions). Some herb–drug interactions are well understood, such as the effect of St John's Wort (used for depression) or grapefruit juice on inhibiting liver breakdown of other drugs (Chan et al., 2010). Warfarin, an anticoagulant, is a western medicine that is quite susceptible to interactions with other western drugs. A recent study of 44 commonly used TCM preparations found that 11 could potentially interact with warfarin in a significant manner (Chua et al., 2015). Unfortunately, many interactions between TCM preparations and drugs are not very clear. Furthermore, western medicine practitioners are often not well versed in the effects and risks of TCM, with the same being true of TCM practitioners.

Given the lack of a pharmacological understanding for many TCMs, postmarketing pharmacovigilance is very important (Xu et al., 2013). China established an adverse drug reaction monitoring system in 1989 that was responsible for reporting on both western

Table 13.2 Safety and quality concerns for TCM preparations

Drug-specific factors	Clinical use factors
Nomenclature: issues include the same name for different herbs and different names for the same plant, which can lead to practitioner or patient confusion	**Lack of theoretical guidance:** TCM drugs should only be used when there is an appropriate TCM diagnosis and the treatment is able to address this condition
Place of origin: plants from designated areas are didao and considered to be of superior quality; differences in growing conditions and climate can lead to different therapeutic effects and interactions	**Drug interactions:** TCMs can interact with western medicines or with other TCMs in a way that can cause significant harm; as the pharmacology of many TCM preparations are not well elucidated, the dangers for drug interactions are even greater
Contamination: plants used in TCM can be contaminated by pesticides, heavy metals or other pollutants	**Adherence failure:** the dosage and timing of many TCMS are based on historical use rather than pharmacokinetics studies; consequently, improper adherence can lead to adverse events through mechanisms that are not well understood
Processing: different processing techniques can lead to different products, which is particularly problematic when processing is important for removing toxic ingredients	**Incorrect drug preparation:** some treatments, such as TCM decoctions, require preparation after purchase; incorrect preparation can lead to decreased efficacy or inadequate removal of toxins
Storage: different storage techniques can lead to deterioration or contamination with bacteria or chemicals	**Storage:** different storage techniques can lead to deterioration or contamination with bacteria or chemicals
Excipients: inactive ingredients can be of low quality, leading to safety concerns for the drug overall	
Manufacturing: GMP and standardized procedures are essential in maintaining drug quality	

Table 13.2 Safety and quality concerns for TCM preparations (continued)

Drug-specific factors	Clinical use factors
Lack of safety studies: often there are insufficient preclinical and clinical data available for TCMs; as a result, postmarketing surveillance is very important	
Counterfeit drugs: intentional counterfeiting or adulteration raises major quality and safety concerns	

Source: Zhang et al., 2012.

and TCM drugs (Zhang et al., 2012). There is a national monitoring centre run by the CFDA along with provincial affiliates that take reports from health care providers, patients and drug manufacturers. TCMs accounted for 13.8% of all adverse drug reaction reports, of which 99.7% were from formulated products and only 0.3% were from crude plants or herbs. TCMs accounted for 12.2% of all serious and unexpected adverse drug reactions (Zhang et al., 2012). Moving forwards, China can improve safety of TCMs by increasing the evidence base behind existing remedies, ensuring Good Agricultural Practice and GMP are adhered to, and strengthening its pharmacovigilance system.

13.5 Export of TCM

The TCM export market is rapidly growing. China's 12th Five Year Plan explicitly sought to increase cooperation with foreign governments and international organizations on the R&D of TCM and to increase international adoption and recognition of TCM (L.E.K., 2012). Meanwhile, consumers in many developed countries are increasingly interested in complementary and alternative therapies, including TCM. The largest export markets are Japan, South Korea and the United States (Songwanich, 2014). Growth in exports of TCM has been quite robust: around 10% for TCM drugs and 12–15% for Chinese herbs (Euromonitor, 2014). The total size of the export market exceeded US$ 2 billion in 2010 and is certainly much higher now (China Chamber of Commerce for Import and Export of Medicine and Health Products, 2011). Many large multinational pharmaceutical companies have taken an interest in TCM and have begun acquiring Chinese forms or engaging in partnership activities. For example, GlaxoSmithKline opened a Discovery Performance Unit in 2012 to apply modern drug-discovery tools to explore TCM, while in 2009 Novartis invested US$ 1 billion opening an R&D centre in Shanghai focusing on R&D including investigation of TCM (L.E.K., 2012).

Increasing use of TCM in western countries has led to concerns about its safety and quality. In Australia, a large study of adverse events from TCM among a broad spectrum of practitioners showed that there was approximately 1 adverse event for every 633 consultations (Bensoussan, Myers & Carlton, 2000). In the United States, the relatively weak regulatory environment for TCM preparations (they are generally considered dietary supplements) has led to calls for increased testing and regulatory control by the US FDA (Ventola, 2010). Some facilities in the United States have detected contaminants such as heavy metals, other medicines and banned chemicals in certain herbal medications (Boyer, 2005).

From a regulatory perspective, the United States allowed TCM to be registered under the US FDA as botanical drugs in 2004. Since then, two – Veregren for the topical treatment of warts and Fulyzaq for the treatment of HIV-associated diarrhoea – have been approved (Wu et al., 2015). Another nine TCM products are in phase II or III clinical trials. In Europe, the European Medicines Agency has allowed herbal medications to be regulated under one of three classes: class I is for traditional use, which has the fewest requirements; class II is for well-established use, which requires scientific evidence for at least ten years along with recognized efficacy and safety; and class III is full market authorization, which requires a full set of clinical data similar to western medicines. There have been approximately 1300 products that have been registered using the relatively simple class I procedure (Wu et al., 2015). The international regulatory environment for TCMs is evolving in order to protect patient safety and to take advantage of exciting new drug development possibilities.

13.6 Conclusions

TCM has been used in China for thousands of years and remains a core component of health care in China. It uses a theoretical understanding of the body and disease that is fundamentally different from the western medicine paradigm. As China has modernized, western medicines have become increasingly popular. However, TCM drugs still account for a substantial proportion of total pharmaceutical sales, particularly in the OTC market. Furthermore, the government is keen to support ongoing R&D of TCM and encourage its export.

There are significant regulatory challenges surrounding TCM. TCM preparations are generally less standardized and often contain a mixture of ingredients. Production must take into account factors such as growing conditions, preparation and storage. Its use is largely based on tradition and history, rather than an understanding of pharmacodynamics and pharmacokinetics. These factors also lead to significant concerns with safety and drug quality. Drug interactions are of particular concern as the mechanisms of action of many TCM preparations are not entirely clear and practitioners often do not have sufficient information.

Many of the challenges facing western drugs are present among TCMs. Reimbursement criteria are not entirely clear and there is a lack of cost–effectiveness or CER; regulation is difficult and there are significant concerns surrounding drug safety. The ever-increasing export market for TCMs means many of these concerns are being transmitted abroad. Moving forwards, the government will need to redouble its efforts to modernize TCM in China. This will involve better quality control, more R&D, clearer and more standardized guidelines on clinical use and better integration into China's increasing western medicine system.

14. Industrial policy

KEY MESSAGES

- China's industrial policy prioritizes building an innovative pharmaceutical sector. However, it is also important that China strengthens its domestic generics industry so it can reliably provide high-quality medications at affordable prices.
- The pharmaceutical industry in China is heavily fragmented, leading to significant quality shortcomings. Local protectionism of weak firms has been a major cause and needs to be overcome.
- Market fragmentation has also meant that China predominantly exports upstream APIs and has largely failed to break out of low-value production. Strengthening the domestic pharmaceutical industry by increasing market concentration is crucial to improving export capabilities.
- Although China is, or will soon be, the world's second largest drug market by total revenue, spending on R&D for innovative products is extremely low by international standards. Furthermore, R&D varies significantly by region, with most of it concentrated in eastern coastal cities and provinces. The government has committed to increased R&D funding, which will be necessary to help to stimulate the industry. Ensuring that this investment leads to effective knowledge diffusion will be important in creating an innovative domestic industry.
- Increased private investment in R&D is also important. Although there are encouraging signs of increased venture capital activity, returns on R&D investment for Chinese companies are currently too low to support an innovative pharmaceutical industry. Raising these returns risks tension with China's other efforts to control drug costs.
- China is still developing its intellectual property laws and should aim to create a system that fosters innovation while minimizing negative consequences such as unnecessary patent battles. Corruption is rife throughout the health care system, and efforts to stamp it out must continue to be encouraged.
- A coordinated national pharmaceutical strategy should incorporate industrial policy goals in order to foster innovation alongside other policy goals of cost-containment, drug quality, affordability and access.

14.1 Chinese pharmaceutical industry in context

Biotechnology is one of the seven priority industries in China's 12th Five Year Plan, with the goal of having life sciences account for at least 4% of China's GDP (KPMG, 2011; Shobert, 2015). While Chinese companies such as Tencent, Alibaba and Lenovo have become global powerhouses, they lack any equivalent in the pharmaceutical industry. The ultimate aim is to shift the pharmaceutical industry up the value chain to become an industry based on innovation rather than low value, low quality production (Hughes, 2010). This will require the achievement of two principal objectives. First, the government must encourage the development of an innovative R&D industry that is capable of developing new drugs. Second, and related, China will need to improve the quality of its generics industry. Both will require higher market concentration and stronger industry standards.

Driven by a combination of economic development and demographic trends, China is already, or soon expected to become, the world's second largest pharmaceutical market (IMS Health, 2013c). The size of China's market gives the Chinese Government a considerable amount of potential influence that can be used to achieve industrial policy objectives (Wang, Chen & Tsai, 2012). The global pharmaceutical market has become increasingly segmented. Industrializing countries such as China have an opportunity to capture elements of the value chain that are currently occupied by multinational corporations (Wang et al., 2012). However, the implementation of industrial policy at a local level is shaped by the huge regional and cultural differences within China. Local governments are often competing and pulling industrial policy in different directions (Bernhardt & Liang, 2014). An interesting comparison can be made between India and China's pharmaceutical industries (Box 14.1).

The fragmentation of the Chinese pharmaceutical industry is well known. This in part stems from competing interests of local governments for regional development and job creation. Rapid development has ensued, but this has been carried out inefficiently, which has led to small-scale, duplicative and low-quality production (Zhou & Lan-Juan, 2013). Small firms are problematic for China's stated high-innovation strategy because their scale prevents them from establishing sufficient profits to fund major R&D investments. They also tend to have a lower level of technology and are less competitive (Chu, Sun & Liang, 2010).

The Chinese Government has recognized that consolidation of its pharmaceutical industry is important. Currently, the Chinese Government requires that any new pharmaceutical manufacturer be "consistent" with national development plans for the industry. This is their response to the concerns that too many pharmaceutical companies are established without sufficiently advanced technology, leading to a waste of resources. By introducing and enforcing international standards of Good Laboratory Practice and GMP it has ensured that only pharmaceutical companies able to afford the technology can survive (Chitour, 2013). By using these standards as a threshold for pharmaceutical companies to survive in the industry, the Chinese Government is able to navigate one of the thorniest

Box 14.1 A comparison of China and India's pharmaceutical industries

India is the largest importer of APIs from China in the world (*The Economic Times*, 2014): 80% of the APIs that India uses comes from China and goes into its robust generic medicines industry. While China is largely unable to export finished drugs and other products higher up the value chain than APIs, India currently produces one third of the world's medicines (Kannan, 2014). This stark contrast in the success of the export industry is interesting considering both India and China are developing countries with a large population and relatively cheap labour force.

In fact, China appears to have the advantages of a better industrial infrastructure, superior and cheaper logistics as well as a very strong education system, particularly in the sciences. However India has promoted its pharmaceutical industry for longer and it is much stronger, with key players who compete in the international market (Zhang, 2012).

Historically, India has more aggressively utilized legal flexibilities within the Trade-Related Aspects of Intellectual Property Rights agreements (Kapczynski, 2009). This enabled India to be more successful than China both in keeping drug prices low for its own population and in ensuring availability of drugs (Li, 2008). The Indian Government has been proactive in asserting its national interest through the introduction of the Drug Price Control Order. India's later implementation of the Trade-Related Aspects of Intellectual Property Rights agreements also does not seem to have harmed its R&D investment or its export capabilities. Indian pharmaceutical companies invest significantly more as a proportion of sales in R&D (Li, 2008). In contrast to China, patents filed in India are mainly from domestic Indian firms (Li, 2008). Indian companies have proved more successful at developing new drug and vaccine candidates and are in advance of China across all stages of the drug development pipeline (Rezaie et al., 2012b).

Indian pharmaceutical companies have been assessed as being more internationally competitive (Li, Yang & Du, 2011). They have managed to grow pharmaceutical exports to over 50% of revenues (Rezaie et al., 2012a). India has over 350 drugs on the WHO's list of prequalified medicinal products for procurement, while China has only 18 (Huang, 2015). In spite of these significant export successes, India has had challenges in creating access to high-quality drugs for its low-income citizens. Consequently, while China can learn from India's export quality standards, it must keep in mind domestic public health goals when moving forwards with overall industrial policy.

China has some way to go before it can catch up with India in terms of generic production or innovative drug development. Nevertheless, it should have the necessary market size and the underlying knowledge substrate to succeed if policies are oriented correctly.

aspects of industrial policy: how to identify "losers" and ensure they wither away to the benefit of "winning" firms (Rodrik, 2004). Evidence from a comprehensive dataset of medium and large enterprises suggests that using industrial policy to foster competition has led to increased productivity growth in the Chinese economy (Harrison et al., 2012). However, interference from local governments interested in protecting local employment and tax bases is rife. By stopping mergers and acquisitions and preventing companies from going out of business, the push for greater consolidation and efficiency is being undermined.

Despite some isolated successes, so far the Chinese pharmaceutical industry has failed to break out of low-value production (Zhang, Cooke & Wu, 2011). The industry is still predominantly focused on APIs and nonproprietary medicines (Li, Yang & Du, 2011). For the majority of pharmaceutical enterprises, R&D spending is less than 5% of sales. Much of this is spent on generics research, further limiting the amounts available for innovative drug development (IBISWorld, 2015c).

Geographically, China's industry is focused in wealthy eastern regions rather than the interior. China's eastern regions have the most firms, the largest share of employees and the highest revenues, profits and exports within the country (Fig. 14.1) (National Bureau of Statistics of China, 2014).

Fig. 14.1 Percentage breakdown of China's pharmaceutical industry by region, 2013

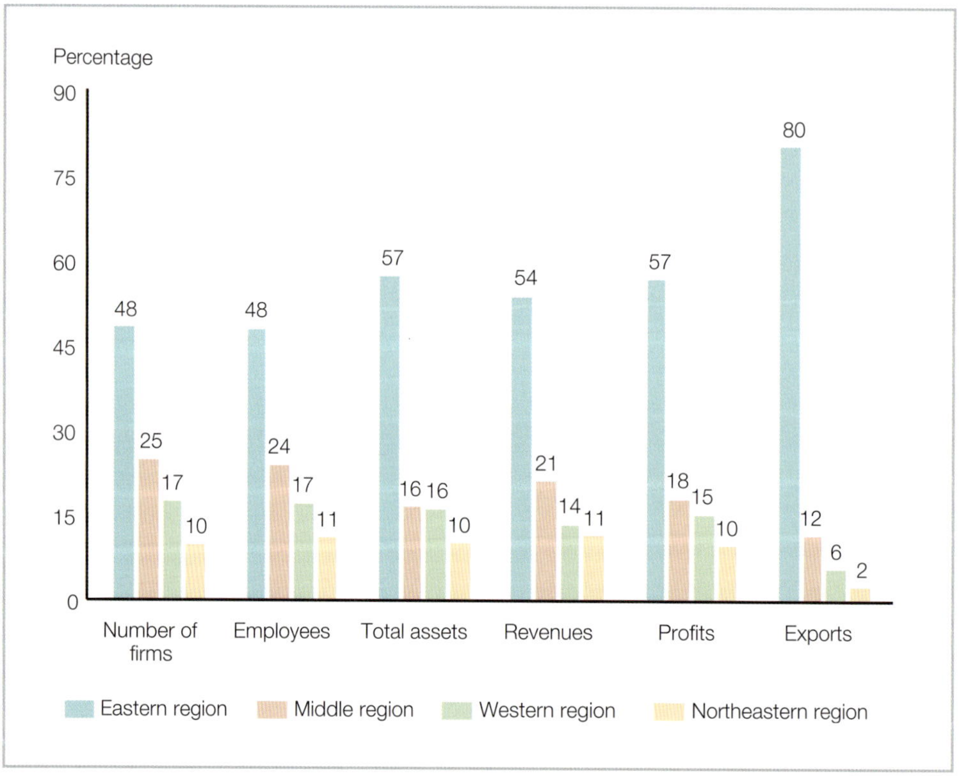

Source: National Bureau of Statistics of China, 2014.

14.2 Components of the Chinese pharmaceutical industry

Production of western medicines can broadly be classified into three categories: APIs, biological and biochemical drugs, and chemical drugs. China is the world leader in the production and export of APIs, the easiest and most upstream product class (Chitour, 2013). Since 2010, revenue from the raw material manufacturing industry has had an average annual growth rate of 15.9% (IBISWorld, 2015d). The majority of revenue for this segment comes from exports, which demonstrates its international competitiveness. As the pharmaceutical raw materials industry does not require high technological capacity, industry profitability is relatively low (IBISWorld, 2015d). Profit margins have been negatively affected by a number of factors such as the appreciation of the yuan renminbi, rising labour costs and increased regulatory costs (IBISWorld, 2015d). Ultimately, the scale of China's industrial ambitions mean that it must diversify from exporting APIs into production of finished drugs.

China has seen strong growth in the biological and biochemical manufacturing industry – an estimated 22.5% per year from 2009 to 2014. The establishment of broader insurance schemes and more public health funding has increased the demand for biological products, particularly vaccines. The government wants to ensure that this industry develops in line with international standards (IBISWorld, 2015a). China's chemical pharmaceutical industry has also experienced solid growth over this period, both in size and in profitability. Revenue for the traditional chemical pharmaceutical industry in China grew by 12.5%, to a total of US$ 107.9 billion in 2014 (IBISWorld, 2015c).

However, both these higher-value segments face a number of challenges. Manufacturing capacity is not well standardized, which leads to excess capacity in times of low demand. A generally weak regulatory and inspection environment can have serious consequences when it comes to drug quality. These problems are exacerbated by low industry concentration: the top five manufacturers in the biological and biochemical sector only have about 20% of total market share. This hinders attempts for China to break out of low-value API exports into the more lucrative generic export market.

Approximately 98% of the pharmaceutical manufacturers in China produce generic drugs (Bernhardt & Liang, 2014). Low-technology generic producers, which compete mostly on price, dominate the Chinese pharmaceutical market. Consequently, margins are low at around 5–10% (IBISWorld, 2015c). Chinese companies dominate sales in the local generic market, while the local innovative drug market is dominated by imports by multinational corporations (Bernhardt & Liang, 2014). State-owned enterprises also tend to focus on the generics market. Their R&D expenditure is remarkably low by international standards, at less than 5% of total revenue (Wang et al., 2012). Exports by domestic firms are very low at only 0.5% of total revenues, which highlights their weakness in terms of international competitiveness.

14.3 Pharmacy industry fragmentation

There are different ways of classifying how many drug manufacturing firms there are in China. Based on the 2013 China Industry Year book, there were 6839 enterprises involved in the manufacture of medicines (National Bureau of Statistics of China, 2014) while the 2013 National Statistics Handbook estimated there were 4629 (Center for Health Statistics and Information, 2013). The top ten pharmaceutical companies in China control less than one fifth of the market, compared with control of about half the market for companies in western countries (Coyne, 2012). Regardless, market fragmentation is a well-recognized problem in China's pharmaceutical environment.

The effects of this fragmentation are profound for the Chinese pharmaceutical industry. The nature of pharmaceutical production, characterized by high capital costs for R&D and expensive production facilities, suggests that a fragmented industry is likely to be duplicative and highly inefficient. As a practical example, in 2004 there were over 20 companies in China that manufactured interferon, with a total production capacity of 400 million bottles. However, actual production was a mere 50 million bottles. Similarly, there were over 100 applications from different companies to market eight commonly prescribed generic medications compounds (CDE, 2015).

There is insufficient regulatory capacity to adequately inspect and monitor such a large number of manufacturers. This allows low cost manufacturers to compete by circumventing already low quality standards, which compromises pharmaceutical safety. The sheer number of companies also creates a significant burden for regulators, which delays their other activities such as approving actually needed medications for patients.

14.3.1 Promoting market concentration

Increasing market concentration is a crucial aspect of improving both the R&D capacity of Chinese firms as well as the quality of generic drug production. The Chinese Government's 12th Five Year Plan explicitly sets the objective of industry consolidation and aims to ensure that the sales of the top 100 enterprises constitute 50% of the total health care industry (Kieger, 2015). This will continue to be a priority in the 13th Five Year Plan, which will span 2016 to 2020. Concentration is very slowly increasing, with the market share of the top 100 firms increasing from less than 40% in 2005 to about 45% in 2013 (Credit Suisse, 2015).

Investors in Chinese firms have traditionally struggled to withdraw their capital gains because of an underdeveloped mergers and acquisition market and strict initial public offering regulations (Qiu et al., 2014). There are signs that this is changing, with the value of deals in the health care sector doubling in 2014 and continuing to accelerate in 2015 (Reuters, 2015). Moreover, the average size of deals has grown significantly, increasing by five times between 2008 and 2013 (Fig. 14.2) (Kieger, 2015).

Fig. 14.2 Merger and acquisition (M&A) deals within China's health care industry, 2008–2013

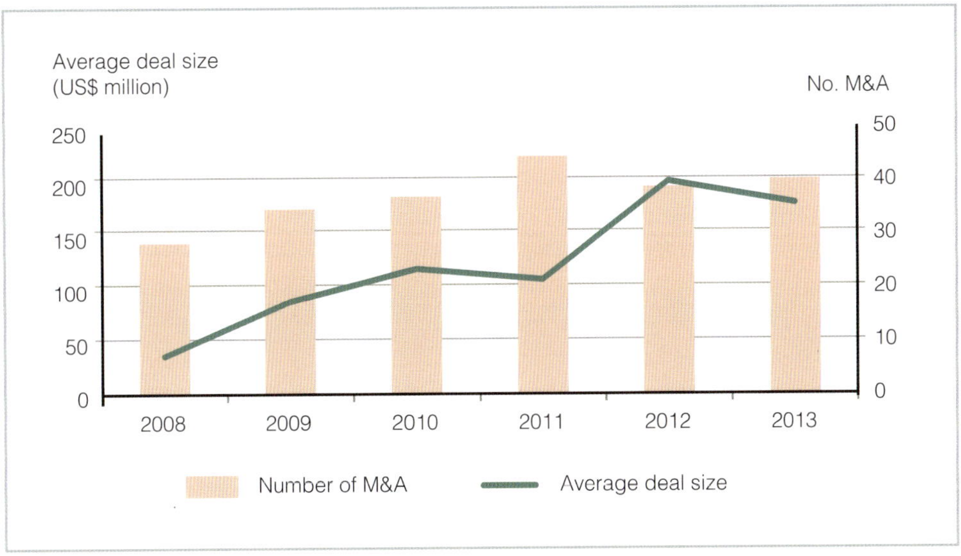

Source: Kieger, 2015.

One of the most significant challenges in achieving greater market concentration has been that local governments sometimes interfere with the closure of poorly performing local enterprises for political reasons (Development Research Center of the State Council, 2015). Local protectionism has been a major barrier to further market consolidation. Many companies provide significant tax revenues for local governments and employment for many workers, so closing them can be very challenging.

Chinese cultural practices can also have implications for the mergers and acquisitions market. Guanxi (personalized networks of influence) is commonplace and means that in practice companies have obligations to other parties because of past relationships that are not shown on financial statements (Coyne, 2012). State-owned enterprises have been known to disguise their "debts" through the invention of transactions between themselves which they have no intention of ever settling (Coyne, 2012).

The government can encourage market consolidation through a number of mechanisms. General policies for encouraging merger and acquisition activity include making financing more easily available for companies seeking to engage in acquisitions and creating a tax environment favourable for mergers and acquisitions. More specific to the pharmaceutical sector, the CFDA has sought to use regulations for Good Laboratory Practice and GMP both to raise the quality of drugs produced in China and to increase market concentration by weeding out weak firms. GMP certification also offers the prize of exports being able to compete better internationally (Macintyre, 2011). The cost of compliance with new standards is likely to have a greater impact on small and medium-sized enterprises (Kieger, 2015). From a drug-procurement perspective, tendering carried out across provinces in order to avoid favouring the companies of any particular region can also help to drive weak manufacturers out of the market. Ultimately, one of the most important policies for encouraging mergers and acquisitions is by withdrawing local protectionism for weak firms.

14.4 R&D

R&D is key to the innovative pharmaceutical industry that the Chinese State wishes to encourage. Despite China having one of the fastest R&D investment growth rates in the world (Chakma et al., 2014), R&D investment as a proportion of GDP remains low and only accounts for 2% of sales, far lower than the 14–18% seen in leading global pharmaceutical companies (Zhou & Lan-Juan, 2013). China also faces challenges from an underdeveloped venture capital system, poor links between research and industry and underperforming intellectual property output (Zhang, Cooke & Wu, 2011). In more developed markets, start-ups contribute considerable innovation to the pharmaceutical value chain, but in China they play a smaller role, partly because of the lack of venture capital investment.

The overall pharmaceutical milieu also contributes to low returns on R&D. A relatively slow approvals process means new drugs take a long time to come to market. When drugs do come to market, pricing policies have been in such flux that pricing is challenging. This, combined with a general lack of attention to drug quality, means that innovative products can potentially be undercut by low-quality products. From a reimbursement perspective, the depth of coverage is low and the NRDL has not been updated in more than half a decade. As a result, even if innovative drugs do come to market many Chinese will not have access to them.

The history of drug R&D in China can be divided into four distinct periods. Initially, Chinese companies simply imitated the synthetic methods and technologies of foreign companies. Over time this progressed to a more innovative form of drug development. Drug innovation came to mean modifying delivery methods and preparation formulae of existing drugs without altering their underlying molecular structure. Eventually China progressed to "imitative innovation". Chemical modifications of existing drugs, such as changing the acid or base group, meant that China was developing "me-too" drugs. The final step of this process, which the Chinese Government is keen to encourage, is the discovery of new chemical entities using advanced technologies (Ding et al., 2011). At each stage, the development of the Chinese pharmaceutical industry was shepherded by relevant regulation, usually from new patent laws. For example, patent law began to give full protection to drugs in 1992 and essentially required that competitors modify molecular structures, which gave rise to "me-too" drugs. This shows the impact government can have on shaping the industry through its choice of regulation.

14.4.1 Public–private mix of investment and geographic variation

China's 12th Five Year Plan aims to increase spending on R&D to 2.2% of GDP (KPMG, 2011). Yet R&D in China, while growing, lags far behind European countries and the United States in terms of pharmaceutical R&D intensity (Fig. 14.3) (Moses et al., 2015). For example, China contributes only 1.8% of the global total towards medical research, in spite of its huge market size (Moses et al., 2015). In 2011, China's R&D intensity was 1.41%, some 17 times lower than in the United Kingdom or the United States (Qiu et al., 2014).

Fig. 14.3 Global medical research funding in selected countries/regions, 2011

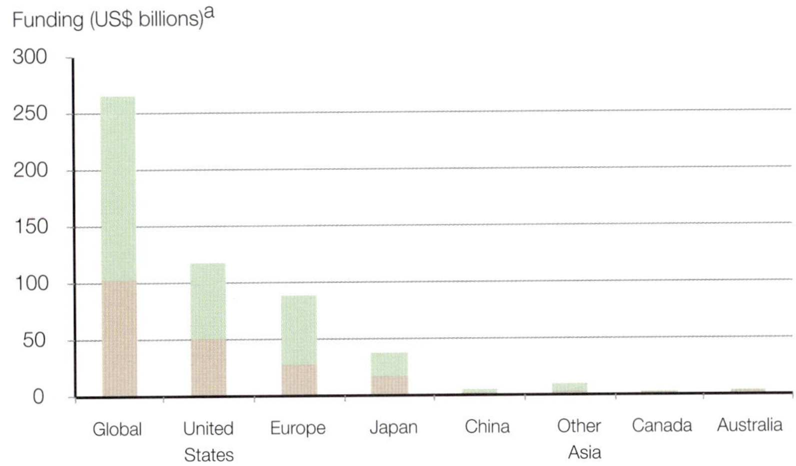

	Global	United States	Europe	Japan	China	Other Asia	Canada	Australia
Overall (US$ billions) (%)	265.0 (100)	117.1 (44)	88.5 (33)	37.8 (14)	4.9 (1.2)	9.7 (4)	3.1 1.2)	3.8 (1.4)
Public[b] (US$ billions) (%)	102.8 (100)	50.5 (49)	26.9 (26)	17.0 (17)	1.3 (2)	2.4 (2)	1.8 (2)	2.8 (3)
Industry[c] (US$ billions) (%)	162.2 (100)	66.6 (41)	61.6 (38)	20.8 (13)	3.6 (0.8)	7.3 (4)	1.3 (0.8)	1.0 (0.6)
Compound annual growth 2004–2011 (%)d	3.5	1.0	4.1	6.8	16.9	20.8	4.5	9.3

Source: Moses et al., 2015.

Notes: [a] Based on an average exchange rate for the year and adjusted to 2012 US dollars using the Biomedical Research and Development Price Index; [b] Includes funding from governmental agencies, higher education institutes and non-profit-making organizations; [c] Pharmaceutical, biotechnology and medical device firms; [d] Calculated based on a rate of x for year A and y for year B using the equation (y/x)[1/(B – A)] – 1; [e] Includes R&D expenditure from 36 major countries from four continents; [f] Includes India, Singapore and South Korea.

Fig. 14.4 Intensity of R&D by region, 2011

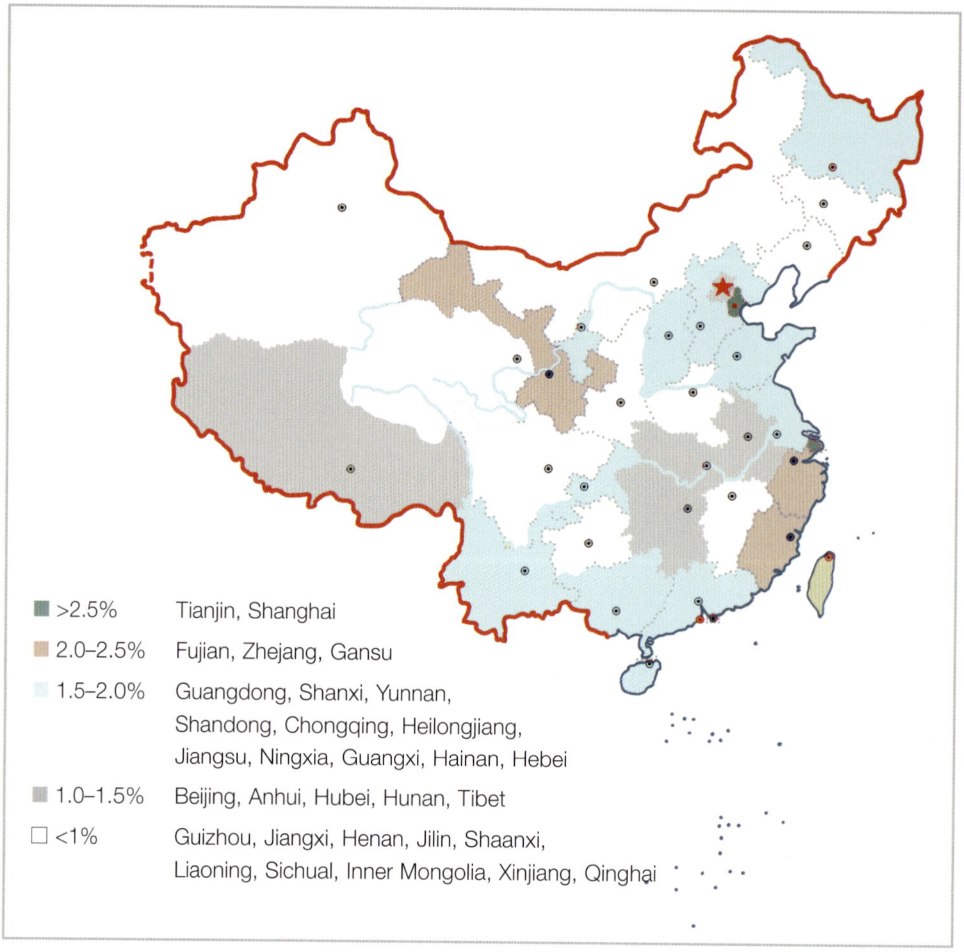

Source: Qiu et al., 2014.

Different areas of the pharmaceutical sector tend to benefit from public and private R&D funding. Public funding is more concentrated in less-developed provinces with substantial natural herbal resources. The TCM and biopharmaceutical subsectors receive more public money than the chemical medicines subsector (Qiu et al., 2014).

There is also significant geographic variation in R&D intensity (Fig. 14.4) (National Bureau of Statistics of China, 2014; Qiu et al., 2014). Some provinces, such as Shandong, Jiangsu and Guangdong, spend far more on R&D than other, particularly western, provinces. As a result, the number of pharmaceutical patent filings is much higher in these provinces (Fig. 14.5) (National Bureau of Statistics of China, 2014). For example, the 10 provinces that file the most patents account for 70% of all patent filings in China (National Bureau of Statistics of China, 2014).

Fig. 14.5 Number of new patent applications of the 10 most productive provinces, 2013

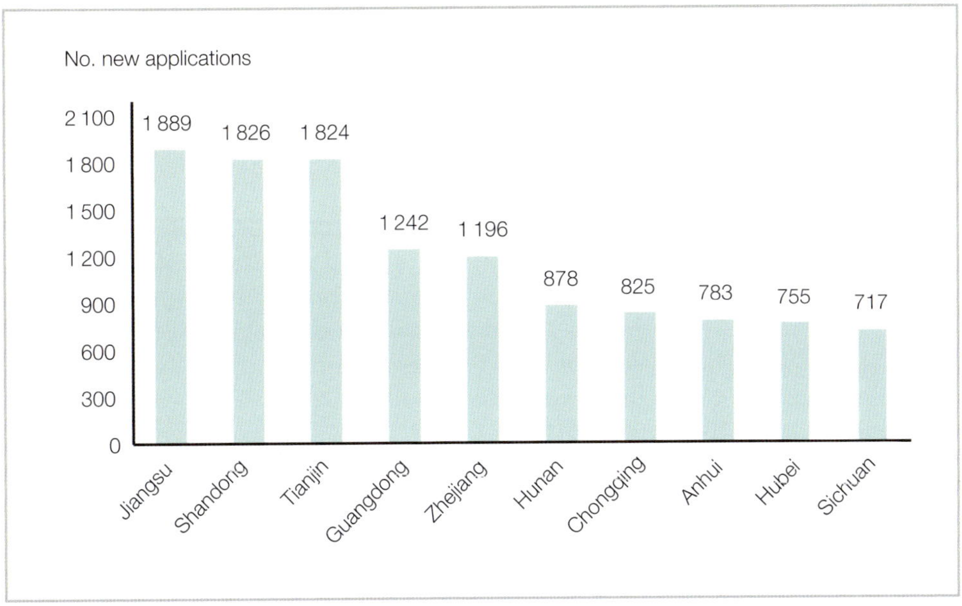

Source: National Bureau of Statistics of China, 2014.

These numbers may even overstate the amount of R&D that is actually taking place in China. Traditionally these statistics convert for purchasing power parity across countries, which may not be appropriate for many components of R&D spending as these are internationally priced (Zhang, Cooke & Wu, 2011). The sustainability of state funding is also debatable (Zhang, Cooke & Wu, 2011).

Private investment is estimated to provide 75% of total pharmaceutical R&D in China (Moses et al., 2015). However, it is unclear how far this R&D money is used to produce genuinely new drugs. Many of the so-called innovative drugs produced are in reality copycat drugs from a clinical perspective (Huang, 2015). There is some evidence to suggest that governmental funding is more important in the development of the most innovative new drugs (Sampat & Lichtenberg, 2011).

It is debatable as to whether China is really reaping the benefits from its investments in R&D. It is true that China has made substantial progress in indicators such as patent applications. In 1991, China filed 1% of global life science patent applications but in 2011 it filed 30% (Moses et al., 2015). However, translation of these figures into a successful home-grown innovative pharmaceutical industry is more tenuous. About half of all inventions in biotechnology are owned by foreign partners (Zhang, Cooke & Wu, 2011). China derives very little of its export revenue from truly innovative products, which is a clear challenge for the pharmaceutical industry in future (Huang, 2015).

14.4.2 Foreign R&D in China

Drugs developed abroad have a more problematic licensing pathway than those developed in China. Following approval abroad, drugs developed overseas are still required to provide local Chinese clinical trial data (Su, 2013). This provides a powerful incentive for international firms to conduct R&D in China initially. In 2008, a new tax law offered preferential income tax rates and turnover tax exemptions to R&D centres providing research services to overseas companies.

China has certainly been successful at moving clinical trials onto its soil. In 2001, only four clinical trials were registered in China, but by 2010 that figure had risen to 497 (Bernhardt & Liang, 2014). China's R&D operations industry has experienced rapid growth, with revenues from the top 10 firms involved in this field rising from RMB 25 billion in 2006 to RMB 63 billion in 2011 (Hvistendahl, 2013). The 20 largest international pharmaceutical companies in the world have all established manufacturing or R&D operations in China (IBISWorld, 2015c).

This success was likely driven by market factors as well as the incentives provided by the Chinese Government. China has a large patient population who are quite willing to be involved in clinical trials. The inclusion of Chinese patients can also be beneficial as word of mouth referral is popular for Chinese consumers (Bernhardt & Liang, 2014). Estimates indicate that clinical trials in China can be conducted between four and ten times faster than in many other industrialized countries, which is clearly attractive for companies looking to market quickly (McTiernan, 2015a).

There are, however, considerable concerns about the reliability and quality of trials conducted in China. GlaxoSmithKline fired its head of R&D in 2013 for misrepresenting data in a clinical trial of an experimental drug for multiple sclerosis (Hvistendahl, 2013). Other drug trials, such as that for the anticoagulant Eliquis (apixaban) have had problems and have on occasion led to delays in US FDA approval (McTiernan, 2015a). If the perception develops that Chinese trials are more likely to be invalid or unacceptable, this could be a significant concern for the research-contracting companies who carry out clinical trials.

Furthermore, there is evidence that higher-level R&D activities are not being moved to China. There seems to be a low level of knowledge diffusion, with multinational corporations merely attracting talent at the expense of local firms because of the higher salaries they can offer (Wang et al., 2012). There is also criticism that the R&D clusters encouraged by state and local governments have resulted in a boom of new science firms that are isolated from domestic state-owned enterprises. Instead, these innovative smaller firms are becoming more closely associated with large multinational corporations (Wang et al., 2012).

14.4.3 High-technology parks and clusters of excellence

China's pharmaceutical industry is concentrated in Beijing, Shanghai, Shenzhen and other major cities. There has been rapid growth in the number of R&D centres in China, which have more than quadrupled since the mid 2000s (Bernhardt & Liang, 2014). These science parks were intended to imitate the Californian Silicon Valley example and build local innovation systems that would coordinate universities, R&D institutes and production units (Wang et al., 2012).

At present, there are approximately 20 relatively mature pharmaceutical clusters in China. While the existence of these bioparks and clusters is a sign of significant investment in pharmaceutical capacity, it remains to be seen whether this number of clusters can be viable in the long term. The danger is that central or local government will be unable to discourage superfluous clusters (Macintyre, 2012).

The government has also sought to encourage relationships between multinational corporations and local firms. Bioparks such as Zhangjiang Park in Shanghai and Zhongguancun Park in Beijing have attracted major international companies such as Eli Lily and Novo Nordisk to establish their R&D headquarters. There is some evidence that these parks have improved research commercialization prospects (Zhang, Cooke & Wu, 2011). The biotechnology parks allow international companies to take advantage of China's many low-wage scientists and smooth the entry of medications into China's market. However, ensuring that China is able to effectively transfer foreign R&D and knowledge to domestic firms still remains a challenge.

14.4.4 Human resources for R&D

The strategic priority for pharmaceutical R&D places substantial demands on China's science workforce. Shortage of talented Chinese employees is one of the greatest challenges to China's pharmaceutical industry (Bernhardt & Liang, 2014). Although China leads the world in terms of the overall size of its science and technology workforce, it has only 1.9 science and technology workers per 10 000 equivalents, which is less than a quarter of that in the United States (Moses et al., 2015). As with other aspects of R&D, human resources are concentrated in a few key provinces (Fig. 14.6) (National Bureau of Statistics of China, 2014). Nevertheless, an estimated 25% of Chinese students who study abroad return to China, which provides a large foreign-trained workforce (Rezaie et al., 2012a).

The Chinese Government has focused on increasing the number of graduates with advanced scientific training using tempting incentives such as increased pay. Whether these students will stay for the longer term is unclear, and there is evidence to suggest that China is not attracting the most highly trained and accomplished group of students to return. There are also suggestions that a large salary gap between international and local staff may harm morale (Hao, 2007). The cost of research scientists in China is still 5–10 times lower than in the United States (Zhang, Cooke & Wu, 2011).

Fig. 14.6 Number of full-time equivalent employees working in R&D by province, 2013

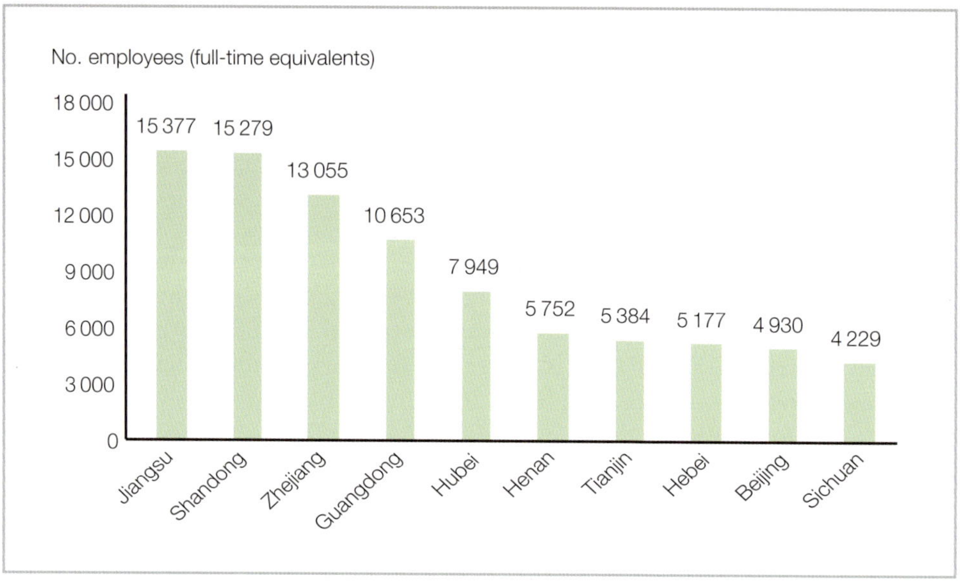

Source: National Bureau of Statistics of China, 2014.

14.5 Intellectual property rights

Intellectual property rights are crucial to the success of a modern pharmaceutical industry. China has established an increasingly comprehensive patent regime that, despite some differences, is similar to what is typically provided under United States or European law (Zhang & Deng, 2008).

The State Intellectual Property Office is the government agency primarily responsible for patents. China first adopted a product patent regime in 1993, at a stage when its pharmaceutical industry was not competitive with developed nations in drug discovery. Patents can be sought for processes and compounds for 20 years but, unlike many other countries, there is no system for patent extension. In principle, there are provisions for drugs containing new chemical entities to gain a five-year market exclusivity period and a six-year data exclusivity period (Wang & Lin, 2014). In practice, concerns have been raised about the actual extent to which data exclusivity is respected and about the loss of patent life through regulatory delays (US-China Economic and Security Review Commission, 2014). In 2012, the State Intellectual Property Office issued a regulation allowing for compulsory licensing in China, although no such licences have ever been issued.

Weaknesses in China's patent system can be seen in other areas. For example, the lack of knowledge of patent infringement can be used as a defence in China. Enforcement of patent legislation can also be problematic; the burden of proof is on the patent holder and legal proceedings must be filed within two years of the date on which the patentee or interested party learned of infringing activities (Zhang & Deng, 2008). Enforcement of intellectual property rights is also decentralized; patent cases are handled by municipal courts in the jurisdiction of the accused, which can lead to potential conflicts of interest (Rezaie et al., 2012a).

China is also experiencing some of the negative impacts that patents can have on innovation. Increasingly, Chinese firms file defensive and offensive patents and are adopting more sophisticated intellectual property strategies. Patents can also be quite politicized, as demonstrated by the example of Viagra in China (Box 14.2). While advanced technical design-around solutions and a generous use of legal challenges are a feature of modern patent systems, they are hardly the productive elements of intellectual property regimes that China should seek to emulate (Zhang & Deng, 2008).

Box 14.2 Viagra's patent in China

Despite the fact that the Viagra patent had been invalidated or revoked in many developed countries such as the United Kingdom, the European Union Patent Office, Australia and Canada, there was considerable controversy in China when its Patent Re-examination Board invalidated the patent (Liu, 2013). China came under heavy criticism from Pfizer, business associations and the United States Government. This politicization of what can be described as a perfectly reasonable decision consistent with other countries' patent decisions probably contributed to the Beijing No. 1 Intermediate People's Court reversing the patent invalidation and allowing the patent protection to be maintained.

Viagra currently holds about 60% of the Chinese market for erectile dysfunction drugs, with a further 20% taken by Eli Lilly's equivalent and a further 10% for Bayer. The current market is estimated at RMB 1 billion annually, but likely has huge untapped potential if prices were to be lowered given that erectile dysfunction affects an estimated 40 million men in China. Fake Viagra has been a considerable problem. When the patent expires, an expected 10 domestic drug-makers will enter the market with generics, which will likely cost about a quarter of the current price (Johnson, 2014). China has, therefore, in this example, somewhat surprisingly ruled in favour of multinational corporations to disadvantage their domestic industry and their patient population. In doing so it has also disagreed with the verdict of several other national patents offices.

14.6 Corruption

Corruption has long plagued the Chinese health care system and until recently had been largely tolerated by the Chinese authorities. Hospital reliance on drug sales and low doctor salaries offer powerful incentives to accept bribes and under-the-table payments are difficult to turn down. The substantial backlog of regulatory drug approvals also creates a potential market for corruption in order to streamline a drug's review. Corruption and bribery may also be contributing to the local protectionism that makes increasing market concentration difficult to achieve. More recently, however, China has taken decisive, if perhaps uneven, action.

In December 2013, the NHFPC issued a prohibition of nine unethical conducts within the health care industry. The prohibition focuses on public health care staff taking or accepting money outside their legitimate income, but also includes prohibitions on participating in marketing exercises, generating statistics for their own organizations (if used for private profit) and procuring drugs not in accordance with legal standards. The anticorruption policy has been placed into key performance indicators for public health care staff, which are vital to their career and promotion prospects (DBS Group Research, 2015).

The recent GlaxoSmithKline scandal also highlighted that the authorities are increasingly willing to act on corruption and that there is a growing trend towards increased government enforcement (Covington and Burling LLP, 2014b). GlaxoSmithKline was hit with the largest bribery fine ever imposed on a foreign company in China, and the company's British head in China received a suspended three-year prison sentence. While these actions have generated headlines, they are seen in many quarters as a symbolic crackdown on dubious practices, with the true motive of reducing drugs prices rather than driving out international pharmaceutical makers (Jia, 2013). GlaxoSmithKline is unlikely to be the only company engaging in these practices given the substantial profits to be made.

These actions in the health care sector form part of President Xi Jinping's wider campaign against corruption in the Chinese Communist Party. Senior officials and even members of the Politburo such as Bo Xilai and Zhou Yongkang have been tried and found guilty of corruption. Despite this increasing and at times dramatic action on corruption, foreign companies have shown no signs of looking to abandon the burgeoning Chinese market (Hvistendahl, 2013). This gives an indication of where the balance of power lies between the international pharmaceutical industry and the Chinese Government. It would suggest that there is scope for increased pressure to be placed on multinational corporations without driving them away. The fact that these corrupt practices are likely to be widespread could also give Chinese authorities leverage over such multinational corporations.

14.7 The 13th Five Year Plan

China has introduced the 13th Five Year Plan, its blueprint for development for 2016 to 2020. Within the Plan there are a number of provisions salient to the health care industry. China has called for significant reforms in drug pricing and quality, health insurance and physician remuneration (Sai, 2015a). There will be a continued push towards increasing market involvement in the determination of drug prices, a move that was initiated with the lifting of price ceilings in the summer of 2015. As outlined by the CFDA and State Council documents early in 2015, improving drug quality will remain a priority. There are also plans for increasing reform and investment in the health insurance systems. This will include merging the URBMI and the NCMS, broader rollout of major disease schemes, greater room for private health insurance and increased government funding for public health insurance. From a provider perspective, there are plans for comprehensive reform of the remuneration of physicians and the medical services industry, likely a reflection of the problems created by the loss of income from the ZMU policy. There will also be further encouragement for the development of primary care, electronic medical records and telemedicine.

China has highlighted its commitment to R&D by designating innovation as one of the guiding principles of the 13th Five Year Plan (PwC, 2015). Medicines and medical devices are one of the ten priority strategic areas that China hopes to foster over the coming five years. Within this, there will be a particular focus on biological products and medical devices (Sai, 2015a). The government also hopes to develop precision medicine – essentially the customization of health care – through technologies such as mobile health, the Internet and Big Data (Wu, 2015). The push for innovation in the pharmaceuticals and medical devices industry will provide opportunities for domestic companies seeking to engage in R&D.

14.8 Conclusions

China is grappling with a dual challenge: how to improve the quality of generics but also support a modern pharmaceutical industry based on R&D and innovation. Increased market concentration will be necessary for both objectives. Higher standards for generics could enable domestic Chinese firms to enter the export market and compete with countries such as India. Higher standards for generics will also be a boon to China's population. As a middle-income country with substantial inequalities, OOP spending and catastrophic health expenditure are major problems that have the potential to cause significant political problems (Li, Liu & Glaetzer, 2013).

China is putting in place the building blocks for a successful pharmaceutical ecosystem based in China, although not necessarily carried out by Chinese companies. Rapid increases in R&D funding form the bedrock of their strategy and have led to increasing numbers of patients and publications. Capital investments in biotechnology parks are welcome. Intellectual property rights have been modernized to close to those in Western countries, although further progress will be needed to foster true innovation. Efforts to eliminate corruption in health care are another important component of rationalizing all aspects of the pharmaceutical environment. Unfortunately, current returns to R&D are still relatively low in China.

While there is a tension between the desire for an innovative pharmaceutical sector that can develop new medications and strengthening the domestic generic sector so that cheap medications can be made broadly available, China has many advantages it can leverage. It has a huge market that is very attractive to domestic and international firms alike, a population that is able to spend more on drugs and an increasing number of foreign-trained graduates returning home with science backgrounds. A coherent national pharmaceutical strategy that incorporates industrial policy will help to promote overall health care goals, particularly as industrial policy is intimately linked with other aspects of policy such as drug regulation and approvals, pricing and reimbursement.

15. Conclusions and policy recommendations

This report has provided an overview of China's past and current pharmaceutical landscape, key issues and challenges and potential opportunities for reform. Rationalizing China's pharmaceutical environment is critical to the success of China's ambitious health care reforms and health improvements for its people. This concluding chapter identifies 11 key areas for improvement and provides specific policy recommendations for reform:

- overall regulatory environment
- drug approvals, drug quality and drug distribution
- key health issues
- affordability and access
- pricing and reimbursement
- prescribing
- hospitals
- primary care
- pharmacies
- TCM
- industrial policy.

It is important to recognize that these pharmaceutical policies are interconnected and that changes should be implemented in a coordinated fashion.

Overall regulatory environment

China's health care and pharmaceutical regulatory environment is highly fragmented. There are many ministries at the national level that wield responsibility; there are also many regional, provincial and local government bodies that play a role in policy development and implementation. Local protectionism is a serious problem that blocks many types of reform, including increasing market concentration and more rational tendering. There is no overarching national pharmaceutical strategy that provides guidance to policy reforms. Corruption is common throughout the health care system and introduces perverse incentives that undermine well-thought-out reforms. Finally, new policies are often not properly evaluated, which makes assessment of their success or failure challenging.

Moving forwards, China should adopt a national pharmaceutical strategy in order to coordinate reform efforts and policy changes. This will allow responsibility for health care delivery and reform to be better harmonized across national ministries and between the national ministries and regional and provincial agencies. Local protectionism should also be addressed in order to encourage market consolidation and improve overall drug quality. Corruption, which is problematic through all sectors in China, should be punished, with licence suspensions and possible criminal consequences for clinicians, bureaucrats and corporations who engage in these practices. Finally, efforts should be made to monitor and evaluate the effects of policy changes in order to inform further reforms.

Drug approvals, quality and distribution

China faces a significant delay in new drug approvals because of the abundance of NDAs from market fragmentation, a lack of effective signalling mechanisms to prioritize approvals (e.g. HTA, CER) and the level of personnel and other capacity at the CFDA. Drug quality is also poor, again stemming from market fragmentation, relatively lax regulatory standards and insufficient CFDA capacity. The drug distribution chain is also highly fragmented, which leads to large price mark-ups between factory and patient use.

It will be important to strengthen the capacity of the CFDA and its provincial affiliates by increasing financial and human resources in order to ensure that drug approvals can be carried out in a timely manner and drug quality can be effectively monitored. Plans for bioequivalence testing for all generic medications as a requirement for approval should be continued and carried out as quickly as possible. Incorporating more CER and HTA into the approval process will be important in guiding and expediting the approval of important drugs while deterring applications for redundant "me-too" generics. Finally, regulatory measures such as stronger GMP and bioequivalence requirements for approval should be used to increase the market concentration for drug manufacturers.

Key health issues

China is facing serious health challenges in the coming decades; its population is rapidly ageing, urbanization has led to unhealthier lifestyles, and environmental degradation and rates of smoking are extremely high. These factors are fuelling a rapid increase in the rate of NCDs such as diabetes, cardiovascular diseases and cancer. The economic burdens associated with this epidemiological transition will also be extremely high.

There are several steps that can improve China's ability to deal with these emerging health challenges. The health system should pivot towards dealing with NCDs on a population level. This means a stronger public health apparatus that engages in preventive activities, health promotion and healthy public policy and regulations. The primary care system should also be strengthened, as it is capable of providing cost-effective and accessible care for NCDs. Specifically from an urbanization perspective, efforts should be made to address the gaps in health care faced by workers migrating to cities as well as to deal with urban environmental degradation through regulations that protect air, water and food quality. Finally, pharmacological management of NCDs is important for health and having a system capable of providing affordable, effective and safe medications for common diseases such as hypertension and diabetes will be crucial.

Affordability and access

In spite of over five years of government reforms, there is still a pervasive perception that health care and pharmaceuticals are not affordable in China. Even though government spending has been accelerating rapidly, OOP expenditure still makes up around 30% of THE. Drug spending makes up about 40% of THE, with many medications, particularly high-quality off-patent originators, being quite expensive. Availability of many essential medications remains tenuous in some regions of China. While insurance coverage is broad, the depth of coverage is low because of high co-payments and deductibles and low reimbursement ceilings. There is significant variation in coverage across the three insurance schemes and geographically, which contributes to significant inequality.

It will be important for insurance coverage to be deepened to decrease co-payments and deductibles. If co-payments must exist, they should be linked to measures of clinical effectiveness (i.e. value-based user charges). Efforts should be made to decrease OOP spending, particularly for vulnerable populations such as poor rural residents and migrant workers and their families. Both equity and efficiency will be enhanced if steps are taken to integrate China's three different insurance schemes. Finally, there must be greater availability of important medicines, particularly EDL drugs, throughout all of China.

Pricing and reimbursement

The 15% mark-up policy has been one of the key drivers of perverse overprescribing in China and is gradually being replaced. Tendering is the dominant pricing mechanism in China but is not sufficiently quality oriented and is beset by challenges with local protectionism. Quality problems have led to huge price gaps between off-patent originators and domestically produced generics. Reimbursement caps are meant to replace price ceilings, but implementation is vague. The two main reimbursement lists, the EDL and the NRDL, have not been updated in three and six years, respectively. Finally, there is little use of HTA or CER in any pricing or reimbursement decisions.

There are a number of ways to rationalize the pricing and reimbursement system. Implementation of the ZMU policy should be continued in order to remove the perverse incentives created by the 15% mark-up. Indeed, any policies that link provider income with prescribing (such as secondary negotiation) should be eliminated. Reforming the tendering process is crucial given its importance. There should be more focus on quality by using objective bioequivalence and GMP data. Steps should also be taken to move towards a more transparent national process in order to promote efficiency and contend with protectionism. Reimbursement caps and guidelines for price negotiations for patented drugs should be made transparently and incorporate CER and HTA as much as possible. Finally, updating reimbursement lists more regularly or even continuously is important to improve access to all medications.

Prescribing

Overprescribing is a huge problem in China, driven by supply-side financial incentives and demand-side patient expectations. Use of antibiotics and injections are far in excess of WHO standards. As a result, China suffers from huge amounts of antibiotic resistance and adverse drug reactions. Drug interactions are another consequence of excessive prescribing. Meanwhile, adherence to medicines for many chronic conditions remains difficult.

To improve the quality of prescribing, financial incentives to prescribe should be eliminated through broader implementation of ZMU, and physician payment reform that rewards quality should be introduced. National campaigns have shown some success at curbing antibiotic use and decreasing antimicrobial resistance and should be continued. Provider education, financial incentives and the use of clinical support systems such as electronic medical records should be encouraged to prevent drug interactions and adverse reactions and to encourage medication adherence. Ideally, such electronic systems would also involve electronic order and entry components and linkages with patient use to be maximally effective. Finally, there should be greater public education on the dangers of medication overuse, particularly in terms of antibiotics and injections, so there is less patient demand for irrational medications.

Hospitals

China is over-reliant on its hospitals for health care provision, even for outpatient services. They account for two thirds of total health care spending and up to 80% of total pharmaceutical spending. Hospitals depend on drug revenue to survive as direct government subsidies are low. Physicians are relatively underpaid and so have an incentive to obtain income through other means such as drug sales and kickbacks. As a result, efforts to remove the link between drug sales and hospital revenues are very challenging. Rollout of ZMU is the most important pharmaceutical policy change related to hospitals. In county hospitals, it has been successful in decreasing hospital reliance on drug sales but lost income has not been compensated by income from other sources. In city hospitals, high-quality evaluation data are lacking.

In general, health system efficiency would be enhanced by shifting service provision from hospitals to primary care and pharmacies. Continuing to remove the link between hospital revenues and drug sales is critical to rationalizing the overall pharmaceutical environment, particularly in urban hospitals where implementation has been limited. Finally, comprehensive payment reform for hospitals and providers is important so that lost drug revenue is replaced, providers are appropriately compensated and quality care rather than prescribing is financially advantageous.

Primary care

China has a weak primary care system. Patients generally prefer to visit hospitals and see specialists for even minor ailments. This is an inefficient way of health care delivery, as primary care can play an important role in high-quality cost-effective care that is focused on prevention. A strong primary care system will be particularly important in managing the increasing rates of NCDs. The EDL and ZMU were first introduced for primary care and have been somewhat effective at improving prescribing and in removing the use of drug revenue to provide care facility revenue. However, the revenue lost from drug sales has not, unfortunately, been replaced by government subsidies and this has led to deficits.

In order to address health care challenges, China should strengthen its primary care system by training more primary care practitioners and increased funding for infrastructure and operations. Integration between hospitals and primary care should be enhanced to allow for better communications and referrals and to improve patient trust in an integrated health care system. Finally, EDL and ZMU should continue to be implemented, but payment reform must address shortfalls in lost drug revenue through higher direct government subsidies, or gaming of the system may occur.

Pharmacies

As with primary care, China has a relatively weak retail pharmacy sector. Unlike almost all western countries, most drugs are sold at hospitals rather than in retail pharmacies. Pharmacists play a limited role in patient education and counselling, nor do they have a strong role in encouraging rational prescribing in inpatient or outpatient settings. China also faces a human resources shortage, particularly in light of regulations that call for newly opened pharmacies to be staffed with licensed pharmacists. Finally, online pharmacies are emerging as an alternative means through which patients can obtain their medications.

Pharmacies offer a promising avenue through which to remove the link between drug sales and hospital revenues and to provide drugs for patients in the community and China should continue with plans to strengthen its pharmacy sector. Pharmacists and clinical pharmacy services should play a larger role in the health care system in terms of patient and provider education on rational prescribing, drug interactions and medication adherence. Increasing training capacity with a focus on clinical pharmacy rather than academic pharmacology and standardizing licensing regulations will be needed to ensure China has enough pharmacists. Online pharmacies represent an exciting alternative to traditional stores but must be monitored and regulated carefully to ensure they are offering safe and affordable medicines.

TCM

Although western medicines are increasing in popularity, TCM continues to be used by a majority of China's population and forms an important part of health care. Regulation and monitoring of the quality of TCM preparations are challenging as they are often mixtures of compounds, are easily prone to contamination, have variable manufacturing processes and their active ingredients are often not known. Interactions with other TCM preparations and western medications pose a significant risk to patients and can be difficult to predict.

As TCMs are such a popular part of health care in China, efforts to modernize the TCM industry should continue. This includes more research on how TCM preparations work, more standardized manufacturing practices, clinical guidelines on their use and so on. Regulations on TCM efficacy and quality should be strengthened in order to ensure that patients are receiving medications that are clinically effective and safe. It is particularly important for there to be robust mechanisms for reporting adverse reactions and drug interactions given the limited understanding of how many TCM preparations work.

Industrial policy

China's pharmaceutical industry faces many challenges. The pharmaceutical industry is generally characterized by market fragmentation, local protectionism and corruption. The generics industry is unable to provide quality medications that are the equal of off-patent originators and China is unable to export chemical drugs competitively. China has also not been successful at building an innovative pharmaceutical sector. R&D spending intensity is much lower than in developed countries as returns on investment for innovation are quite low. In spite of attracting significant interest from multinational corporations because of the size of the Chinese market, it is not clear that significant knowledge diffusion is occurring.

Improving the industrial policy environment is a key priority of the Chinese Government and is embedded within its 13th Five Year Plan. Moving forwards, it will be important to focus on both increasing innovative R&D activities and ensuring that there is a robust generics industry capable of producing affordable, high-quality medications. Increasing market concentration is crucial for both the domestic generics industry and innovative R&D. This can be done through fighting local protectionism, strengthening GMP and quality standards and creating an environment conducive to mergers and acquisitions. Further increases in R&D spending are needed to create an innovative pharmaceutical industry. This will require not only direct government funding but also the creation of a policy environment conducive to higher returns on research (e.g. faster drug approvals, better reimbursement coverage, a focus on quality).

As one of the world's largest pharmaceutical markets, China can leverage foreign interest and knowledge to develop its own research capacity. Finally, as with kickbacks and bribes at the clinician or hospital level, corruption at the level of drug companies must be punished severely to ensure a level playing field for all competitors.

15.1 Summary

China has a complex pharmaceutical environment that is undergoing significant reforms as part of a broader effort to improve health care. There are a number of challenges with the current system. Pharmaceutical spending makes up almost 40% of all health care spending and has been growing rapidly over recent years. Unfortunately, drug revenues still account for a large percentage of hospital and physician income through the 15% mark-up policy. This has encouraged significant amounts of irrational prescribing and problems with antibiotic and injection overuse. Fragmentation in drug manufacturing and distribution have led to high drug prices and problems with drug quality. The government has made progress in expanding the population covered by insurance but many gaps remain, with low coverage ceilings and high deductibles for many medicines. The hospital system is highly entrenched and powerful while public health, primary care and pharmacies are relatively weak. From a regulatory perspective, CFDA regulations have not been strict enough nor has its capacity for oversight been strong enough to create a quality supply of medications. Industrial policy has been lacking, leading to weakness in the manufacturing of generic domestics and home-grown innovation. Finally, problems with local protectionism, corruption and a lack of transparency have limited the effectiveness of many reform efforts. Fortunately, the government has recognized the need for significant system-level reforms for rationalizing the pharmaceutical system.

In 2014 and 2015, a large number of reforms were introduced in the areas of pricing and reimbursement, drug quality and physician and hospital payment reform, and these are moving China in the right direction. These reforms include the ZMU policy, quality-based tendering, a greater emphasis on CER and HTA, and higher drug quality standards. From a broader health system perspective, it is commendable that the government is strengthening primary care and pharmacies in order to better address health care needs characterized increasingly by NCDs in an ageing population. While the pace of reform has been rapid, it is important to recognize that reforming a system that provides health care for 1.3 billion people will take years if not decades. Moving forwards, it will be important to monitor and evaluate the effects of reforms in order to decide which policies to continue. Adopting a national pharmaceutical strategy that takes into account the myriad challenges and opportunities will lend greater coherency to efforts in reforming both the pharmaceutical sector and the overall health care system. While much work still needs to done, continuing on the path of reform will help to guarantee that all Chinese citizens will eventually have access to safe, effective and high-quality medications.

References

11ey.com (2015). *NDRC: 442 drug-price complaints in June.* (http://www.11ey.com/archives/43853.html, accessed 10 March 2016; in Chinese).

Abel-Smith B, Grandjeat P (1978). *Pharmaceutical consumption.* Brussels, Commission of the European Communities.

Academy of Macroeconomic Research (2015). *NDRC: approaching reimbursement caps.* Beijing, Academy of Macroeconomic Research of the National Development and Reform Commission (http://article.haoxiana.com/193989.html, accessed 10 March 2016; in Chinese).

Alcorn T, Ouyang Y (2012). Diabetes saps health and wealth from China's rise. *Lancet,* 379(9833):2227–2228.

Alliance for Safe Online Pharmacies (2015). *The Chinese internet pharmacy market.* Washington, DC, Alliance for Safe Online Pharmacies.

Anderson K (2013). *General and personal medical services: England 2002–2912.* Leeds, NHS Health and Social Care Information Centre (http://www.hscic.gov.uk/catalogue/PUB09536/nhs-staf-2002-2012-gene-prac-rep.pdf, accessed 10 March 2016).

Audit Commission (1995). *The doctor's tale: the work of hospital doctors in England and Wales.* London: HMSO.

Bao L, Peng R, Wang Y, Ma R, Ren X, Meng W et al. (2015). Significant reduction of antibiotic consumption and patients' costs after an action plan in China, 2010–2014. *PLOS ONE,* 10(3), e0118868.

Barber N (1995). What constitutes good prescribing? *British Medical Journal,* 310(6984):923–925.

Barber SL, Yao L (2010). *Health insurance systems in China: a briefing note.* Geneva, World Health Organization (World Health Report 2010 Background Paper 37) (http://www.who.int/healthsystems/topics/financing/healthreport/37ChinaB_YFINAL.pdf, accessed 10 March 2016).

Barber SL, Huang B, Santoso B, Laing R, Paris V, Wu C (2013). The reform of the essential medicines system in China: a comprehensive approach to universal coverage. *Journal of Global Health,* 3(1):010303.

Barber SL, Borowitz M, Bekedam H, Ma J (2014). The hospital of the future in China: China's reform of public hospitals and trends from industrialized countries. *Health Policy and Planning*, 29(3):367–378.

Beam C (2014). Under the knife. *The New Yorker*, August 25 (http://www.newyorker.com/magazine/2014/08/25/under-the-knife, accessed 10 March 2016).

Bensoussan A, Myers SP, Carlton AL (2000). Risks associated with the practice of traditional Chinese medicine: an Australian study. *Archives of Family Medicine*, 9(10):1071–1078.

Bernhardt P, Liang Y (2014). *Challenges, opportunities, and strategies for foreign pharmaceutical MNCs in China: a case study of Bayer Health Care in China* [MA thesis]. Aarhus, Aarhus University (http://pure.au.dk/portal-asb-student/files/76744303/MASTER_THESIS_Bernhardt_Liang_mainbody.pdf, accessed 10 March 2016).

Bhattacharyya O, Delu Y, Wong ST, Bowen C (2011). Evolution of primary care in China 1997–2009. *Health Policy*, 100(2–3):174–180.

Bloom D, Cafiero E, McGovern M, Prettner K, Stanciole A, Weiss J et al. (2013). *The economic impact of non-communicable disease in China and India: estimates, projections, and comparisons*. Cambridge, MA, National Bureau of Economic Research (NBER Working Paper No. 19335) (http://www.nber.org/papers/w19335, accessed 10 March 2016).

BloombergBusiness (2015). Why the FDA is worried about chinese drugs in your medicine cabinet. *Bloomberg News*, October 28 (http://www.bloomberg.com/news/articles/2015-10-28/fda-shows-up-a-man-runs-and-questions-emerge-on-china-s-drugs, accessed 10 March 2016).

Blumenthal D, Hsiao W (2005). Privatization and its discontents: the evolving Chinese health care system. *New England Journal of Medicine*, 353(11):1165–1170.

BMI Research (2015). *Russia pharmaceuticals & healthcare report*. London, BMI Research.

Boston Consulting Group (2014). *New rules for winning in China's pharmaceutical market*. Hong Kong, Boston Consulting Group.

Boyer EW (2005). Issues in the management of dietary supplement use among hospitalized patients. *Journal of Medical Toxicology*, 1(1):30–34.

Brown MT, Bussell JK (2011). Medication adherence: WHO cares? *Mayo Clinic Proceedings*, 86(4):304–314.

Brown R, Piriz D, Liu Y, Moore J (2012). *Reforming health care in China: historical, economic, and comparative perspectives.* Ann Arbor, MI, Gerald R. Ford School of Public Policy at the University of Michigan (PUBPOL 716) (http://sites.fordschool.umich.edu/china-policy/files/2012/07/PP_716_Final_Policy_Paper_Health-Final.pdf, accessed 10 March 2016).

Carone G, Schwierz C, Xavier A (2012). *Cost-containment policies in public pharmaceutical spending in the EU.* Brussels, European Commission (Economic Papers 461) (http://ec.europa.eu/economy_finance/publications/economic_paper/2012/pdf/ecp_461_en.pdf, accessed 10 March 2016).

CDE (2015). 2014 *Annual report on drug review.* Beijing, Center for Drug Evaluation of China Food and Drug Administration.

Center for Health Statistics and Information (2013). *China health statistical handbook.* Beijing, Center for Health Statistics and Information.

Center for Health Statistics and Information (2014). *China health statistical handbook.* Beijing, Center for Health Statistics and Information.

CFDA (2015a). *Reform plan for registration categories of chemical drugs.* Beijing, China Food and Drug Administration.

CFDA (2015b). *Soliciting public opinions regarding policies to expedite the reduction of drug registration application backlog.* Beijing, China Food and Drug Administration (Document 140).

Chakma J, Sun GH, Steinberg JD, Sammut SM, Jagsi R (2014). Asia's Ascent: global trends in biomedical R&D expenditures. *New England Journal of Medicine,* 370(1):3–6.

Chan E, Tan M, Xin J, Sudarsanam S, Johnson DE (2010). Interactions between traditional Chinese medicines and western therapeutics. *Current Opinion in Drug Discovery & Development,* 13(1):50–65.

Chan KW (2012). Migration and development in China: trends, geography and current issues. *Migration and Development,* 1:37–41.

Chee G, Xie Z, Nakhimovsky S (2012). *Evaluation of GAVI-Government of China hepatitis B vaccination program.* Geneva, GAVI (http://www.gavi.org/results/evaluations/evaluation-of-the-gavi-government-of-china-hepatitis-b-vaccination-programme/, accessed 10 March 2016).

Chen M, Wang L, Chen W, Zhang L, Jiang H, Mao W (2014). Does economic incentive matter for rational use of medicine? China's experience from the essential medicines program. *PharmacoEconomics,* 32(3):245–255.

Chen Y, Yin Z, Xie Q (2014). Suggestions to ameliorate the inequity in urban/rural allocation of healthcare resources in China. *International Journal for Equity in Health*, 13(1):34.

Chen Z (2009). Launch of the health-care reform plan in China. *Lancet*, 373(9672):1322–1324.

Chen Z (2012). Early results of China's historic health reforms: the view from Minister Chen Zhu. Interview by Tsung-Mei Cheng. *Health Affairs*, 31(11):2536–2544.

Chen Z, Peto R, Zhou M, Iona A, Smith M, Yang L et al. (2015). Contrasting male and female trends in tobacco-attributed mortality in China: evidence from successive nationwide prospective cohort studies. *Lancet*, 386(10002):1447–1456.

Cheng W, Fang Y, Fan D, Sun J, Shi X, Li J (2012). Study on the effect of "zero mark-up" policy on medicines in Beijing community health facilities. *Pharmaceuticals Policy and Law*, 14:177–186.

Cheung F (2011). TCM: made in China. *Nature*, 480(7378), S82–S83.

China CDC (2012). *China national plan for NCD prevention and treatment (2012–2015).* Beijing, China Centre for Disease Control and Prevention (http://www.chinacdc.cn/en/ne/201207/t20120725_64430.html, accessed 7 March 2016).

China Chamber of Commerce for Import and Export of Medicine and Health Products (2011). *Top 20 export markets of traditional Chinese medicines 2010*. Beijing, China Chamber of Commerce for Import and Export of Medicine and Health Products (http://www.cccmhpie.org.cn/Pub/3737/25545.shtml, accessed 10 March 2016).

China Nonprescription Medicines Association (2012). *Blue paper on OTC industry development in China*. Beijing, China Nonprescription Medicines Association.

Chitour H-L (2013). Big pharma in China: the driving forces behind their success – a qualitative analysis. *Chinese Studies*, 2(4):169–177.

Christiansen A (2014). More than 2000 Chinese students caught cheating on national pharmacist test. *PBS Newshour*, October 29 (http://www.pbs.org/newshour/rundown/2000-chinese-students-caught-cheating-national-pharmacist-test/, accessed 10 March 2016).

Chu S, Sun C, Liang C (2010). Pharmaceutical enterprises' R&D strategic alliance: the road for small and medium sized pharmaceutical enterprises' R&D in China. *International Business Research*, 131–136.

Chua YT, Ang XL, Zhong XM, Khoo KS (2015). Interaction between warfarin and Chinese herbal medicines. *Singapore Medical Journal*, 56(1):11–18.

Covington (2013). *CFDA releases draft revision of primary drug approval regulation.* Beijing, China Food and Drug Administration.

Covington and Burling LLP (2014a). *CFDA release draft measures on unannounced pharmaceutical drug inspections.* Beijing, Covington and Burling LLP.

Covington and Burling LLP (2014b). *Chinese Government ministries issue opinion on implementing pharmaceutical reform.* Beijing, Covington and Burling LLP.

Coyne C (2012). A comparison of the financial characteristics of pharmaceutical firms in the United States and the People's Republic of China. *International Research Journal of Applied Finance*, 3(7):940–953.

CPA-McKinsey (2015). *CPA-McKinsey China hospital pharmaceuticals report: an in-depth perspective.* Beijing, CPA-McKinsey.

Credit Suisse (2015). *China chemical drug sector.* Hong Kong, Credit Suisse.

Currie J, Lin W, Meng J (2014). Addressing antibiotic abuse in China: an experimental audit study. *Journal of Development Economics*, 110:39–51.

Currie J, Lin W, Zhang W (2011). Patient knowledge and antibiotic abuse: evidence from an audit study in China. *Journal of Health Economics*, 30(5):933–949.

Daemmrich A (2013). The political economy of healthcare reform in China: negotiating public and private. *SpringerPlus*, 2(1):448.

Dai H, Fang L, Malouin R, Huang L, Yokosawa K, Liu G (2013). Family medicine training in China. *Family Medicine*, 45(5):341–344.

DBS Group Research (2015). *China healthcare sector: concentrated Chinese medicine granule.* Hong Kong, DBS Group Research.

De Broe ME (2012). Chinese herbs nephropathy and Balkan endemic nephropathy: toward a single entity, aristolochic acid nephropathy. *Kidney International*, 81(6):513–515.

Deloitte (2011). 2011 *Survey of health care consumers in China.* Shanghai, Deloitte Center for Health Solutions.

Deloitte (2015). 2015 *Life sciences outlook Brazil.* Sao Paulo, Deloitte Brazil.

Development Research Center of the State Council (2014). *Development Research Centre joint seminars.* Beijing, Development Research Center of the State Council.

Development Research Center of the State Council (2015). *Development Research Centre joint seminars*. Beijing, Development Research Center of the State Council.

Ding J, Xue Y, Liang H, Shao R, Chen Y (2011). From imitation to innovation: a study of China's drug R&D and relevant national policies. *Journal of Technology, Management and Innovation*, 6(2):1–13.

Dong H, Bogg L, Rehnberg C, Diwan V (1999). Drug policy in China: pharmaceutical distribution in rural areas. *Social Science and Medicine*, 48(6):777–786.

Dong L, Yan H, Wang D (2011). Drug prescribing indicators in village health clinics across 10 provinces of Western China. *Family Practice*, 28(1):63–67.

Dukes G, Haaijer F, de Joncheere C, Rietveld A, eds. (2003). *Drugs and money: prices, affordability and cost containment*, 7th edn. Amsterdam, IOS Press for the World Health Organization.

Edney A (2014). Drug quality in China still poses risks for US market. *Bloomberg News*, April 4 (http://www.bloomberg.com/news/articles/2014-04-03/drug-quality-in-china-still-poses-risks-for-u-s-market, accessed 10 March 2016).

Ellis S (2015). *China's "zero markup" hospital reforms mixed bag for patented drugs*. Atlanta, GA, BioWorld (http://www.bioworld.com/content/chinas-zero-markup-hospital-reforms-mixed-bag-patented-drugs-2, accessed 20 March 2016).

Euromonitor (2014). *TCM industry overview*. London, Euromonitor.

Fang Y (2014). China should curb non-prescription use of antibiotics in the community. *British Medical Journal*, 348(1), g4233–g4233.

Fang Y (2015). Pharmaceutical pricing policies in China. In: Babar Z-U-D, ed. *Pharmaceutical prices in the 21st century*. New York, Springer:43–58.

Fang Y, Yang S, Feng B, Ni Y, Zhang K (2011). Pharmacists' perception of pharmaceutical care in community pharmacy: a questionnaire survey in Northwest China. *Health and Social Care in the Community*, 19(2):189–197.

Fang Y, Yang S, Zhou S, Jiang M, Liu J (2013). Community pharmacy practice in China: past, present and future. *International Journal of Clinical Pharmacy*, 35(4):520–528.

Fudong A, Boyang Y (2011). The status and prospects of the licensed pharmacist qualification system in China. *European Journal of Business and Management*, 3(5):3–6.

Fugh-Berman A (2000). Herb–drug interactions. *Lancet*, 355(9198):134–138.

Ge S, He T-T, Hu H (2014). Popularity and customer preferences for over-the-counter Chinese medicines perceived by community pharmacists in Shanghai and Guangzhou: a questionnaire survey study. *Chinese Medicine*, 9(1):22.

Gong P, Liang S, Carlton EJ, Jiang Q, Wu J, Wang L et al. (2012). Urbanisation and health in China. *Lancet*, 379(9818):843–852.

Gu D, Reynolds K, Duan X, Xin X, Chen J, Wu X et al. (2003). Prevalence of diabetes and impaired fasting glucose in the Chinese adult population: International Collaborative Study of Cardiovascular Disease in Asia (InterASIA). *Diabetologia*, 46(9):1190–1198.

Guan X, Liang H, Xue Y, Shi L (2011). An analysis of China's national essential medicines policy. *Journal of Public Health Policy*, 32(3):305–319.

Guangdong Provincial HFPC (2012). *Notice regarding health care institutions' prescription formulary management*. Guangzhou, Guangdong Provincial BHFPC (http://www.gdwst.gov.cn/a/yzcyaowuzhengce/2013110811044.html, accessed 10 March 2016; in Chinese).

Han S, Liang H, Su W, Xue Y, Shi L (2013). Can price controls reduce pharmaceutical expenses? A case study of antibacterial expenditures in 12 Chinese hospitals from 1996 to 2005. *International Journal of Health Services*, 43(1):91–103.

Hao X (2007). Review: a European-inspired renaissance for China's drug industry. Even oil optimists expect energy demand to outstrip supply. *Science*, 317:436–437.

Harney A (2014). Dearth of doctors drags on China private healthcare drive. *Reuters Business*, October 6 (http://uk.reuters.com/article/china-healthcare-private-idUKL3N0RR2WC20141006, accessed 10 March 2016).

Harrison A, Legros P, Du L, Aghion P, Dewatripont M (2012). *Industrial policy and competition*. Cambridge, MA, National Bureau of Economic Research (NBER Working Paper 18048) (http://www.nber.org/papers/w18048.pdf, accessed 10 March 2016).

Harrison M, Yao J (2014). China healthcare: taking the private route. *KPMG Our View*, December (https://www.kpmg.com/CN/en/IssuesAndInsights/ArticlesPublications/Newsletters/Our-View/Documents/Our-View-1412-05-taking-the-private-route.pdf, accessed 10 March 2016).

He JA (2011). China's ongoing public hospital reform: initiatives, constraints and prospect. *Journal of Asian Public Policy*, 4(3):342–349.

He W, James SA, Merli MG, Zheng H (2014). An increasing socioeconomic gap in childhood overweight and obesity in China. *American Journal of Public Health*, 104(1), e14–e22.

Heddini A, Cars O, Qiang S, Tomson G (2009). Antibiotic resistance in China: a major future challenge. *Lancet*, 373(9657):30.

Hirschler B, Jourdan A (2015). China rejects 11 drug applications over inadequate trial data. *Reuters Markets*, November 12 (http://www.reuters.com/article/2015/11/12/us-china-pharmaceuticals-idUSKCN0T11FZ20151112#T6LaT7shS73vB6Mc.97, accessed 10 March 2016).

Hsiao W, Li M, Zhang S (2014). *Universal health coverage: the case of China*. Geneva, United Nations Research Institute for Social Development (Paper 15).

Hu M, Yee G, Zhou N, Yang N, Jiang X (2014). Development and current status of clinical pharmacy education in China, *American Journal of Pharmaceutical Education*, 78(8):157.

Hu S (2013). Essential medicine policy in China: pros and cons. *Journal of Medical Economics*, 16(2):289–294.

Hu S, Zhang Y, He J, Du L, Xu M, Xie C et al. (2015). A case study of pharmaceutical pricing in China: setting the price for off-patent originators. *Applied Health Economics and Health Policy*, 13(Suppl 1):13–20.

Huang Y (2015). *Chinese pharma: a global health game changer?* Washington, DC, Council on Foreign Relations (http://www.cfr.org/china/chinese-pharma-global-health-game-changer/p36365, accessed 10 March 2016).

Hufeng W (2013). *In-depth analysis of public hospital reform: pilot evaluation*. Beijing, Renmin University Health Reform and Development Centre.

Hughes B (2010). China spurs pharma innovation. *Nature Reviews: Drug Discovery*, 9(8):581–582.

Hvistendahl M (2013). Drug development. Corruption and research fraud send big chill through big pharma in China. *Science*, 341(6145):445–446.

IBISWorld (2015a). *Biological and biochemical product manufacturing in China*. Beijing, IBISWorld (Industry Report).

IBISWorld (2015b). *Pharmacies and drugstores in China*. Beijing, IBISWorld (Industry Report).

IBISWorld (2015c). *Pharmaceutical manufacturing in China*. Beijing, IBISWorld (Industry Report).

IBISWorld (2015d). *Pharmaceutical raw material manufacturing in China*. Beijing, IBISWorld (Industry Report).

IMS Health (2013a). *China: IMS pharmaceutical pricing and reimbursement concise guide*. London, IMS Health.

IMS Health (2013b). *Exploring impacts of the revised EDL and associated policies*. Shanghai, IMS Health.

IMS Health (2013c). *Pharmerging markets*. London, IMS Health.

IMS Health (2013d). *The global use of medicines: outlook through* 2017. London, IMS Health.

IMS Health (2014a). *IMS market prognosis: China*. London, IMS Health.

IMS Health (2014b). *Research report on establishing an optimal reimbursement system in china*. Beijing, IMS Health.

IMS Health (2015a). *Global medicines use in* 2020. London, IMS Health.

IMS Health (2015b). *Vision for a healthier China: proposal for a patient-centred health-care system*. Beijing, IMS Health.

Institute of Economic Research (2014). *The current status, existing problems and reform recommendations of China's pharmaceutical production and distribution system*. Beijing, National Development and Reform Commission.

Institute of Medicine (2000). *To err is human: building a safer health system*. Washington, DC, Institute of Medicine.

Institute of Medicine (2006). *Preventing medication errors*. Washington, DC, Institute of Medicine.

Jacobzone S (2000). *Pharmaceutical policies in OECD countries: reconciling social and industrial goals*. Paris, Organisation for Economic Co-operation and Development (Labour Market and Social Policy Occasional Paper 40).

Jia H (2013). China clampdown on GSK linked to drug costs. *Nature Biotechnology*, 31(10):861.

Jia W (2014). Diabetes? A challenge for China in the 21st century. *Lancet Diabetes Endocrinology*, 2(4), e6–e7.

Jiang J (2011). Patents: protecting China's national treasure. *Nature*, 480(7378), S93–S93.

Jiang M, Yang S, Yan K, Liu J, Zhao J, Fang Y (2013). Measuring access to medicines: a survey of prices, availability and affordability in Shaanxi province of China. *PLOS ONE*, 8(8).

Jiang M, Zhou Z, Wu L, Shen Q, Lv B, Wang X et al. (2014). Medicine prices, availability, and affordability in the Shaanxi Province in China: implications for the future. *International Journal of Clinical Pharmacy*, 37(1):12–17.

Jiang Q, Yu BN, Ying G, Liao J, Gan H, Blanchard J et al. (2012). Outpatient prescription practices in rural township health centers in Sichuan Province, China. *BMC Health Services Research*, 12(1):324.

Jiang Y, Xu Y, Bi Y, Wang L, Zhang M, Zhou M et al. (2015). Prevalence and trends in overweight and obesity among Chinese adults in 2004–10: data from three nationwide surveys in China. *Lancet*, 386, S77.

Johnson E (2014). China pharma industry rises to the occasion as Viagra patent expires. *The Street*, October 6 (http://www.thestreet.com/story/12739816/1/china-pharma-industry-rises-to-the-occasion-as-viagra-patent-expires.html, accessed 10 March 2016).

Jourdan A (2015). China to allow online sales of prescription drugs as early as this month: sources. *Reuters Life*, January 9 (http://www.reuters.com/article/2015/01/09/us-china-pharmaceuticals-idUSKBN0KI0Y220150109?utm_source=The+Sinocism+China+Newsletter&utm_campaign=cda0ebd3cf-Sinocism01_11_15&utm_medium=email&utm_term=0_171f237867-cda0ebd3cf-29593965&mc_cid=cda0ebd3cf&mc_eid=, accessed 10 March 2016).

Kanavos P, Taylor D (2007). Pharmacy discounts on generic medicines in France: is there room for further efficiency savings? *Current Medical Research and Opinion*, 23(10):2467–2476.

Kanavos P, Seeley L, Vandoros S (2009). *Tender systems for outpatient pharmaceuticals in the European Union*. London, London School of Economics (http://ec.europa.eu/health/files/docs/study_pricing_2007/tendering_systems_en.pdf, accessed 10 March 2016).

Kannan S (2014). India "too reliant" on Chinese drug imports, worries Delhi. *BBC News*, December 5 (http://www.bbc.com/news/business-30330898, accessed 10 March 2016).

Kapczynski A (2009). Harmonization and its discontents: a case study of TRIPS implementation in India's pharmaceutical sector. *California Law Review*, 97(6):1571–1649.

Kennedy-Martin T, Mitchell BD, Boye KS, Chen W, Curtis BH, Flynn JA et al. (2014). The health technology assessment environment in mainland China, Japan, South Korea, and Taiwan: implications for the evaluation of diabetes mellitus therapies. *Value in Health Regional Issues*, 3:108–116.

Kieger (2015). *Healthcare in China*. Zurich, Kieger (www.kieger.com, accessed 7 March 2016).

KPMG (2011). *China's 12th five year plan: overview*. Beijing, KPMG China (http://www.kpmg.com/cn/en/IssuesAndInsights/ArticlesPublications/Documents/China-12th-Five-Year-Plan-Overview-201104.pdf, accessed 10 March 2016).

Lancet Editorial (2012). Ending violence against doctors in China. *Lancet*, 379(9828):1764.

Leape LL, Bates DW, Cullen DJ, Cooper J, Demonaco HJ, Gallivan T et al. (1995). Systems analysis of adverse drug events. ADE Prevention Study Group. *Journal of the American Medical Association*, 274(1):35–43.

Lee GKY, Wang HHX, Liu KQL, Cheung Y, Morisky DE, Wong MCS (2013). Determinants of medication adherence to antihypertensive medications among a Chinese population using Morisky Medication Adherence Scale. *PLOS ONE*, 8(4), e62775.

L.E.K. (2012). *Globalization of traditional Chinese medicine (TCM)*. Shanghai, L.E.K.

Li B, Adab P, Cheng KK (2015). The role of grandparents in childhood obesity in China: evidence from a mixed methods study. *International Journal of Behavioral Nutrition and Physical Activity*, 12(1):91.

Li C (2012). *The political mapping of China's tobacco industry and anti-smoking campaign*. Washington, DC, Brookings Institute (China Center Monograph 5).

Li D, Yang C, Du Q (2011). On the value chain and international specialization of China's pharmaceutical industry. *Journal of International Commerce and Economics*, 3:81–107.

Li H, Liu GG, Glaetzer C (2013). Financing innovative medicines in mainland China: the role of commercial health insurance. *Chinese Studies*, 2(3):128–133.

Li J-S, Zhang X-G, Wang H-Q, Wang Y, Wang J-M, Shao Q-D (2013). The meaningful use of EMR in Chinese hospitals: a case study on curbing antibiotic abuse. *Journal of Medical Systems*, 37(2):9937.

Li X (2008). The impact of higher standards in patent protection for pharmaceutical industries under the TRIPS agreement: a comparative study of China and India. *World Economy*, 31(10):1367–1382.

Li X, Huo H, Kong W, Li F, Wang J (2014). Physicians' perceptions and attitudes toward clinical pharmacy services in urban general hospitals in China. *International Journal of Clinical Pharmacy*, 36(2):443–450.

Li Y (2014). China's misuse of antibiotics should be curbed. *British Medical Journal*, 348, g1083.

Li Y, Xu J, Wang F, Wang B, Liu L, Hou W et al. (2012). Overprescribing in China, driven by financial incentives, results in very high use of antibiotics, injections, and corticosteroids. *Health Affairs*, 31(5):1075–1082.

Li Y, Ying C, Sufang G, Brant P, Bin L, Hipgrave D (2013). Evaluation, in three provinces, of the introduction and impact of China's national essential medicines scheme. *Bulletin of the World Health Organization*, 91:184–194.

Li Z, Hou J, Lu L, Tang S, Ma J (2012). On residents' satisfaction with community health services after health care system reform in Shanghai, China, 2011. *BMC Public Health*, 12(Suppl 1), S9.

Liao Q, Lv T, Qiao Y, Wang J (2015). Clinical development of investigational new drug. In: Lu MQ, ed. *Approaching China's pharmaceutical market: a fundamental guide to clinical drug development.* New York, Springer:467–506.

Lim L (2014). Beijing's "Airpocalypse" spurs pollution controls, public pressure. *npr*, March (http://www.npr.org/2013/01/14/169305324/beijings-air-quality-reaches-hazardous-levels, accessed 10 March 2016).

Liu Q, Wang B, Kong Y, Cheng K (2011). China's primary health-care reform. *Lancet*, 377(9783):2064–2066.

Liu Y (2013). The tale of Viagra patents: comparative studies of the global challenges in China and other countries. *Journal of Intellectual Property Rights*, 18:523–533.

Liu Y-Y, Wang Y, Walsh TR, Yi L-X, Zhang R, Spencer J et al. (2015). Emergence of plasmid-mediated colistin resistance mechanism MCR-1 in animals and human beings in China: a microbiological and molecular biological study. *Lancet Infectious Diseases*, 16(2):161–168.

Long Q, Xu L, Bekedam H, Tang S (2013). Changes in health expenditures in China in 2000s: has the health system reform improved affordability. *International Journal for Equity in Health*, 12(1):40.

Lopez Bastida J, Mossialos E (2000). Pharmaceutical expenditure in Spain: cost and control. *International Journal of Health Services*, 30(3):597–616.

Ma D, Adams W (2013). *In line behind a billion people.* Upper Saddle River, NJ, FT Press.

Macintyre BM (2011). Raising the bar: new GMP clears competitive landscape. *CPB Review*, 54:39–43.

Macintyre BM (2012). Localizing discovery. *CPB Review*, 65:21–24.

Mao W, Vu H, Xie Z, Chen W, Tang S (2015). Systematic review on irrational use of medicines in China and Vietnam. *PLOS ONE*, 10(3), e0117710.

Masseria C, Irwin R, Thomson S, Gemmill M, Mossialos E (2009). *Primary care in Europe*. Brussels, European Commission.

Mattke S, Liu H, Hunter LE, Gu K, Newberry S (2014). *The role of health care transformation for the Chinese dream*. Boston: RAND Health.

McKinsey (2010). *China health care reforms*. Shanghai, McKinsey.

McKinsey (2012). *Private health insurance in China: finding the winning formula*. Shanghai, McKinsey.

McKinsey (2014). *India pharma* 2020. Mumbai, McKinsey.

McTiernan R (2014a). Au revoir to Anhui: China's shape-shifting tenders. *CPB Review*, 85:20–25.

McTiernan R (2014b). E-retailing: Alibaba or the forty thieves? *CPB Review*, 82:24–28.

McTiernan R (2014c). Regulatory infarction: CFDA clogs new drug pipeline. *CPB Review*, 87:18–23.

McTiernan BR (2015a). Exploring China's clinical trial value chain SMOs and hospital interactions, *CPB Review*, 88:22–26.

McTiernan R (2015b). Picking a path: CDE debuts biosimilars guidelines. *CPB Review*, 90:18–22.

McTiernan R (2015c). Pipe dreams: CDE offers dose of realism on DAL, DRR reforms. *CPB Review*, 92:20–24.

McTiernan R (2015d). Pricing play: NDRC reveals "liberalization" hand. *CPB Review*, 89:18–22.

Meng Q, Cheng G, Silver L, Sun X, Rehnberg C, Tomson G (2005). The impact of China's retail drug price control policy on hospital expenditures: a case study in two Shandong hospitals. *Health Policy and Planning*, 20(3):185–196.

Meng Q, Xu L, Zhang Y, Qian J, Cai M, Xin Y et al. (2012). Trends in access to health services and financial protection in China between 2003 and 2011: a cross-sectional study. *Lancet*, 379(9818):805–814.

Meng Q, Yang H, Chen W, Sun Q, Liu X (2015). People's Republic of China: health system review. *Health Systems in Transition*, 5:1–246.

Miller LH, Su X (2011). Artemisinin: discovery from the Chinese herbal garden. *Cell*, 146(6):855–858.

Ministry of Health (1989). *General hospital tier management and standards draft*. Beijing, Ministry of Health (http://wenku.baidu.com/link?url=8KNTbkJ8hP5qalU-o4KD-uj6LAM4kAWq21H-sVl57_24XcjLjgbpEUY10LosaCC_Bg33kdAt-YzHhK7DavweWJjgy10-aTeLlslsK41mDLa, accessed 10 March 2016; in Chinese).

Ministry of Health (2010). *Hospital prescription review management (pilot)*. Beijing, Ministry of Health (http://www.china.com.cn/policy/txt/2010-03/04/content_19518502.htm, accessed 10 March 2016; in Chinese).

Ministry of Health (2011a). *Notice regarding tertiary general hospital evaluation criteria*. Beijing, Ministry of Health (http://www.nhfpc.gov.cn/yzygj/s3585u/201112/06f754a213d8413787904e9e6439d88b.shtml, accessed 10 March 2016; in Chinese).

Ministry of Health (2011b). *Progress and achievements of public hospital reform pilots*. Beijing, Ministry of Health (http://www.gov.cn/gzdt/2011-03/21/content_1828888.htm, accessed 10 March 2016; in Chinese).

Ministry of Health, State Commission Office for Public Sector Reform, NDRC, Ministry of Finance, Ministry of Human Resources and Social Security (2010). *Guidance on public hospital pilot reforms*. Beijing, National Health and Family Planning Commission (http://www.gov.cn/ztzl/ygzt/content_1661148.htm, accessed 10 March 2016; in Chinese).

Moses H, Matheson DHM, Cairns-Smith S, George BP, Palisch C, Dorsey ER (2015). The anatomy of medical research. *Journal of the American Medical Association*, 313(2):174.

Mossialos E, Mrazek M, Walley T (2004). *Regulating pharmaceuticals in Europe: striving for efficiency, equity and quality*. Milton Keynes, UK, Open University Press.

Mossialos E, Oliver A (2005). An overview of pharmaceutical policy in four countries: France, Germany, the Netherlands and the United Kingdom. *International Journal of Health Planning and Management*, 20(4):291–306.

Mou J, Cheng J, Zhang D, Jiang H, Lin L, Griffiths SM (2009). Health care utilisation amongst Shenzhen migrant workers: does being insured make a difference? *BMC Health Services Research*, 9:214.

Mou J, Griffiths SM, Fong H, Dawes MG (2013). Health of China's rural-urban migrants and their families: a review of literature from 2000 to 2012. *British Medical Bulletin*, 106(1):19–43.

National Bureau of Statistics of China (2014). *China statistics yearbook on high technology industry*. Beijing, National Bureau of Statistics.

National Bureau of Statistics of China (2015). *National data*. Beijing, National Bureau of Statistics (http://data.stats.gov.cn/english/, accessed 10 March 2016).

National Health Development Research Center (2013). *China national health accounts report*. Beijing, National Health Development Research Center.

National People's Congress (2015). *Decision of the National People's Congress on authorizing the State Council to carry out the pilot programs for the drug marketing authorization holder system in some regions and relevant issues*. Beijing, National People's Congress.

NDRC (2014a). *Notice of the National Development and Reform Commission (NDRC) on enhancing supervision on drug market pricing activities*. Beijing, National Development and Reform Commission (Document 930).

NDRC (2014b). *The current status, existing problems and reform recommendations of China's pharmaceutical production and distribution system*. Beijing, National Development and Reform Commission.

NDRC (2015). *Improving the monitoring of drug prices*. Beijing, National Development and Reform Commission (Discussion Paper).

NDRC, NHFPC, Ministry of Human Resources and Social Security (2014). *Notice regarding the issue of using market regulation to adjust prices for non-public hospitals*. Beijing, National Development and Reform Commission, National Health and Family Planning Commission and Ministry of Human Resources and Social Security (http://www.mohrss.gov.cn/gkml/xxgk/201404/t20140422_128933.htm, accessed 10 March 2016; in Chinese).

Ngai C (2014). Drug procurement and pricing in China. In: *4th Asia Pacific Pharmaceutical Congress, Shanghai 17 September*. Shanghai, Baker & McKenzie (http://www.ehcca.com/presentations/asianpharma4/ngai_ms9.pdf, accessed 10 March 2016).

Ngorsuraches S, Meng W, Kim BY, Kulsomboon V (2012). Drug reimbursement decision-making in Thailand, China, and South Korea. *Value in Health*, 15(1), S120–S125.

NHFPC (2013a). *Prohibition on 9 unethical conducts to strengthen morals in the healthcare industry.* Beijing, National Health and Family Planning Commission.

NHFPC (2013b). *Report on assessment of county-level hospital general reform pilots.* Beijing, National Health and Family Planning Commission (http://www.ahyg.gov.cn/showNews.asp?newsID=3432, accessed 16 March 2016; in Chinese).

NHFPC (2013c). *Several opinions on accelerating the development of medical institutions established by social capital.* Beijing, National Health and Family Planning Commission (http://www.moh.gov.cn/tigs/wslgf/201401/239ae12d249c4e38a5e2de457ee20253.shtml, accessed 10 March 2016; in Chinese).

NHFPC (2014a). *National plan for medical and health services (2015–2020).* Beijing, National Health and Family Planning Commission (http://www.nhfpc.gov.cn/guihuaxxs/s3586s/201410/bbfdb9306fe54da492b6f7d1d64ab8d3.shtml, accessed 10 March 2016; in Chinese).

NHFPC (2014b). *Notice regarding the second round of public hospital reform nationally designated pilot cities and related work plan.* Beijing, National Health and Family Planning Commission (http://www.nhfpc.gov.cn/tigs/s3581/201405/e16bc82c70594c26902454fc97c7ec76.shtml, accessed 10 March 2016; in Chinese).

NHFPC (2014c). *Opinions on multi-site physician practice (draft).* Beijing, National Health and Family Planning Commission (http://www.nhfpc.gov.cn/yzygj/s3578/201401/f5c7c83dffbf4f859c271913131ed958.shtml, accessed 10 March 2016; in Chinese).

NHFPC (2015). *Implementing and improving centralized bidding and procurement of drugs* Beijing, National Health and Family Planning Commission (Document 70) (http://www.moh.gov.cn/yaozs/s3573/201506/36a74780403d4eed96ca93b665620941.shtml, accessed 10 March 2016; in Chinese).

Niu L (2015). *Healthcare in China: A Kieger report on the Chinese healthcare market.* Zurich, Kieger.

OECD (2013a). *Health at a glance 2013: OECD indicators.* Paris, Organisation for Economic Co-operation and Development (http://www.oecd.org/els/health-systems/Health-at-a-Glance-2013.pdf, accessed 10 March 2016).

OECD (2013b). Pharmaceutical generic market share. In: *Health at a glance 2013: OECD indicators.* Paris, Organisation for Economic Co-operation and Development:104–105.

OECD (2014b). *Health statistics: how does China compare?* Paris, Organisation for Economic Co-operation and Development (http://www.oecd.org/els/health-systems/Briefing-Note-CHINA-2014.pdf, accessed 10 March 2016).

OECD (2015a). *Health at a glance 2015: OECD indicators*. Paris, Organisation for Economic Co-operation and Development.

OECD (2015b). Pharmaceutical spending trends and future challenges. In: *Health at a glance 2015: OECD indicators.* Paris, Organisation for Economic Co-operation and Development:29–43.

Oortwijn W, Mathijssen J, Banta D (2010). The role of health technology assessment on pharmaceutical reimbursement in selected middle-income countries. *Health Policy*, 95(2-3):174–184.

Pan XR, Yang WY, Li GW, Liu J (1997). Prevalence of diabetes and its risk factors in China, 1994. National Diabetes Prevention and Control Cooperative Group. *Diabetes Care*, 20(11):1664–1669.

Penm J, Li Y, Zhai S, Hu Y, Chaar B, Moles R (2013). The impact of clinical pharmacy services in China on the quality use of medicines: a systematic review in context of China's current healthcare reform. *Health Policy and Planning*, September, 1–24.

Penm J, Moles R, Wang H, Li Y, Chaar B (2014). Factors affecting the implementation of clinical pharmacy services in China. *Qualitative Health Research*, 24(3):345–356.

Pharmnet (2015). *Perspective on new tendering platforms in three provinces: will drug prices collapse?* (http://news.pharmnet.com.cn/news/2015/07/09/423811.html).

Philipsen NJ (2013). Regulation of pharmacists: a comparative law and economics analysis. *European Journal of Comparative Economics*, 10(2):225–241.

PhRMA (2015). The Prescription Drug User Fee Act (PDUFA) VI. Washington, DC, PhRMA (http://www.phrma.org/pdufa, accessed 10 March 2016).

PPD (2013). *Optimizing drug registration in China: category I route.* Wilmington, NC, Pharmaceutical Product Development (http://www.ppdi.com/drug-registration-china/China_CategoryI-Registration-PPD_White%20Paper.pdf, accessed 10 March 2016).

Press Trust of India (2014). 2440 Chinese students caught cheating pharmacy license test. *Business Standard*, October 27 (http://www.business-standard.com/article/pti-stories/2440-chinese-students-caught-cheating-pharmacy-license-test-114102700645_1.html, accessed 10 March 2016).

PR Newswire (2015). China Jo-Jo announces further healthcare reform by PRC's State Council. *PR Newswire* (http://www.prnewswire.com/news-releases/china-jo-jo-announces-further-healthcare-reform-by-prcs-state-council-300166831.html, accessed 10 March 2016).

PwC (2015). *Prosperity for the masses by 2020.* Beijing, PwC (http://www.pwchk.com/home/eng/prosperity_masses_2020.html, accessed 10 March 2016).

Qi M (2012). The analysis of Chinese drug safety supervision and management. *Chinese Law and Government*, 45(2):3–8.

Qiu J (2015). When the East meets the West: the future of traditional Chinese medicine in the 21st century. *National Science Review*, 2(3):377–380.

Qiu L, Chen Z-Y, Lu D-Y, Hu H, Wang Y-T (2014). Public funding and private investment for R&D: a survey in China's pharmaceutical industry. *Health Research Policy and Systems*, 12(1):27.

qqjjsj.com (2015). *2015 Chinese public health funding increased from 35 to 40 RMB per person* (http://www.qqjjsj.com/zgjjdt/53519.html, accessed 10 March 2016; in Chinese).

Raschetti R, Morgutti M, Menniti-Ippolito F, Belisari A, Rossignoli A, Longhini P et al. (1999). Suspected adverse drug events requiring emergency department visits or hospital admissions. *European Journal of Clinical Pharmacology*, 54(12):959–963.

Reuters (2015). China drug approval backlog jumped by a third last year. *Reuters Life*, March 13 (http://www.reuters.com/article/2015/03/13/us-china-pharmaceuticals-idUSKBN0M90QP20150313, accessed 10 March 2016).

Reynolds L, McKee M (2011). Serve the people or close the sale? Profit-driven overuse of injections and infusions in China's market-based healthcare system. *International Journal of Health Planning and Management*, 26(4):449–470.

Rezaie R, McGahan AM, Frew SE, Daar AS, Singer PA (2012a). Emergence of bio-pharmaceutical innovators in China, India, Brazil, and South Africa as global competitors and collaborators. *Health Research Policy and Systems*, 10(1):18.

Rezaie R, McGahan AM, Daar AS, Singer PA (2012b). Innovative drugs and vaccines in China, India and Brazil. *Nature Biotechnology*, 30(10):923–926.

Rizzi SJ, Lin M (2011). *Generic drug approval process in China.* New York, Food and Drug Law Institute.

Rodrik D (2004). *Industrial policy for the twenty-first century.* Cambridge, MA, Harvard University Press (https://www.sss.ias.edu/files/pdfs/Rodrik/Research/industrial-policy-twenty-first-century.pdf, accessed 10 March 2016).

Rohde RA, Muller RA (2015). Air pollution in China: mapping of concentrations and sources. *PLOS ONE*, 10(8), e0135749.

Roland Berger (2014). *Entering China's private hospital segment.* Beijing, Roland Berger (https://www.rolandberger.com/media/pdf/Roland_Berger_TAB_Entering_Chinas_private_hospital_segment_20140530.pdf, accessed 10 March 2016).

Sai B (2015a). *General trends of healthcare aspects of the 13th five year plan.* Beijing, pharmacy.hc360.com (http://info.pharmacy.hc360.com/2015/11/040855580108.shtml, accessed 10 March 2016; in Chinese).

Sai B (2015b). *Jiangsu drug tender: large price increases.* Prague, PharmNet (http://news.pharmnet.com.cn/news/2015/12/01/433314.html, accessed 10 March 2016; in Chinese).

Sai B (2015c). *NHFPC: transparent tendering and secondary negotiations.* Beijing, pharmacy.hc360.com (http://info.pharmacy.hc360.com/2015/10/220858577827.shtml, accessed 10 March 2016; in Chinese).

Sampat BN, Lichtenberg FR (2011). What are the respective roles of the public and private sectors in pharmaceutical innovation? *Health Affairs (Project Hope)*, 30(2):332–339.

Shen J, Sun Q, Zhou X, Wei Y, Qi Y, Zhu J et al. (2011a). Pharmacist interventions on antibiotic use in inpatients with respiratory tract infections in a Chinese hospital. *International Journal of Clinical Pharmacy*, 33(6):929–933.

Shen JJ, Wang Y, Lin F, Lu J, Moseley CB, Sun M et al. (2011b). Trends of increase in western medical services in traditional medicine hospitals in China. *BMC Health Services Research*, 11:212.

Shi L, Yang HY, Cheng G, Meng Q (2014). Time trends and determinants of pharmaceutical expenditure in China (1990–2009). *PharmacoEconomics*, 32(3):257–264.

Shobert B (2015). Will Apple's business model work in pharmaceuticals? *Forbes*, March 11 (http://www.forbes.com/sites/benjaminshobert/2015/03/11/will-apples-business-model-work-in-pharmaceuticals/, accessed 10 March 2016).

Song P, Li W, Zhou Q (2014). An outpatient antibacterial stewardship intervention during the journey to JCI accreditation. *BMC Pharmacology and Toxicology*, 15(1):8.

Song Y, Bian Y, Petzold M, Li L, Yin A (2014a). Effects of the National Essential Medicine System in reducing drug prices: an empirical study in four Chinese provinces. *Journal of Pharmaceutical Policy and Practice*, 7(1):12.

Song Y, Bian Y, Petzold M, Li L, Yin A (2014b). The impact of China's national essential medicine system on improving rational drug use in primary health care facilities: an empirical study in four provinces. *BMC Health Services Research*, 14(507):1–7.

Songwanich S (2014). The value of traditional Chinese medicine. *The Nation*, March 11 (http://www.nationmultimedia.com/opinion/The-Value-of-traditional-Chinese-medicine-30232325.html, accessed 10 March 2016).

Starfield B, Shi L, Macinko J (2005). Contribution of primary care to health systems and health. *Milbank Quarterly*, 83(3):457–502.

State Council (2009). *Opinions of the CPC Central Committee and the State Council on deepening the health care system reform*. Beijing, State Council (http://www.china.org.cn/government/scio-press-conferences/2009-04/09/content_17575378.htm, accessed 10 March 2016).

State Council (2012a). *12th five year plan on drug safety and standards*. Beijing, State Council.

State Council (2012b). *Notification by the State Council on issuing of program and implementation plan of deepening health system reform in the period of the 12th five year plan*. Beijing, State Council (Notification No.11.).

State Council (2014). *State Council Working Group report on deepening health system reform*. Beijing, State Council (Document 67) (http://www.nhfpc.gov.cn/tigs/ygjb/201412/6c14736455e649ffaf4c9d27e7ca6773.shtml, accessed 10 March 2016; in Chinese).

State Council (2015a). *Guidelines of the General Office of the State Council for the pilot comprehensive reform of urban public hospitals*. Beijing, State Council.

State Council (2015b). *Implementing and improving centralized bidding and procurement of drugs*. Beijing, State Council (Document 7)

State Council (2015c). *Opinions of the State Council on reforming the evaluation and approval system for drugs and medical devices*. Beijing, State Council (Document 44).

State Council (2015d). *State Council healthcare reform 2015 work plan*. Beijing, State Council.

State Council (2015e). *State Council national healthcare service system plan (2015–2020)*. Beijing, State Council (http://www.gov.cn/zhengce/content/2015-03/30/content_9560.htm, accessed 10 March 2016; in Chinese).

State Council (2015f). *State Council organisation chart.* Beijing, State Council (http://english.gov.cn/state_council/2014/09/03/content_281474985533579.htm, accessed 10 March 2016).

Su L (2013). Drug development models in China and the impact on multinational pharmaceutical corporations. *Food and Drug Law Institute Update,* September/October, 19–23.

Sun C, Chai W, Zhou Y, Wang Y (2014). Medicine and surgery challenges facing China's public health and primary health care in health care reform. *Journal of Vascular Medicine and Surgery,* 2(2):8–11.

Sun J (2013). International experiences of promoting generics use and its implications to China. *Journal of Evidence-Based Medicine,* 6(2):74–80.

Sun Q, Santoro MA, Meng Q, Liu C, Eggleston K (2008). Pharmaceutical policy in China. *Health Affairs,* 27(4):1042–1050.

Sun Y (2007). *The situation on GMP and regulatory compliance for APIs manufactured in China.* Beijing, Beijing CHNMED Pharmaceutical Consulting.

Swinburn BA, Sacks G, Hall KD, McPherson K, Finegood DT, Moodie ML et al. (2011). The global obesity pandemic: shaped by global drivers and local environments. *Lancet,* 378(9793):804–814.

Tang Y, Zhang X, Yang C, Yang L, Wang H, Zhang X (2013). Application of propensity scores to estimate the association between government subsidy and injection use in primary health care institutions in China. *BMC Health Services Research,* 13(1):183.

Tang Y, Zhao M, Wang Y, Gong Y, Yin X, Zhao A et al. (2015). Non-adherence to anti-tuberculosis treatment among internal migrants with pulmonary tuberculosis in Shenzhen, China: a cross-sectional study. *BMC Public Health,* 15(1):474.

Tao J, Zhang T, Xu J, Wu C (2013). Analysis of the current situation of antibiotics use in China: a hospital-based perspective. *Therapeutic Innovation and Regulatory Science,* 47(1):23–31.

Tatlow DK (2013). Chinese doctors becoming targets of patients' anger. *Sinosphere,* November 1 (http://sinosphere.blogs.nytimes.com/2013/11/01/doctors-the-targets-of-patients-anger/?_r=0.

The Economic Times (2014). China should open up to Indian generic drugs: experts. *The Economic Times,* September 16 (http://articles.economictimes.indiatimes.com/2014-09-16/news/53983182_ 1_indian-companies-indian-pharmaceutical-apis, accessed 7 March 2016).

The Economist (2014b). Physician, heal thyself: medicines are over-prescribed and over-priced. *The Economist,* February 1 (http://www.economist.com/news/china/21595431-medicines-are-over-prescribed-and-overpriced-physician-heal-thyself, accessed 20 March 2016).

The Economist (2012). Violence against doctors: heartless attacks. *The Economist,* July 21 (http://www.economist.com/node/21559377, accessed 7 March 2016).

The Economist (2014a). Government coughers. *The Economist,* February 27 (http://www.economist.com/news/china/21597958-smoking-course-kill-100m-chinese-people-century-will-latest-anti-smoking, accessed 7 March 2016).

The Wall Street Journal (2015). Falling through the cracks of China's health care system. *The Wall Street Journal,* January 4 (http://www.wsj.com/articles/falling-through-the-cracks-of-chinas-health-care-system-1420420231, accessed 7 March 2016).

Thomson S, Schang L, Chernew ME (2013). Value-based cost sharing in the United States and elsewhere can increase patients' use of high-value goods and services. *Health Affairs*, 32(4):704–712.

Tian X, Song Y, Zhang X (2012). National essential medicines list and policy practice: a case study of China's health care reform. *BMC Health Services Research*, 2009:12:401.

Tordoff JM, Norris PT, Reith DM (2008). "Price management" and its impact on hospital pharmaceutical expenditure and the availability of medicines in New Zealand hospitals. *Value in Health*, 11(7):1214–1226.

Tse E, Pan P, Sun S, Ma K (2012). *Changing landscape of China's pharmaceutical distribution industry.* Beijing, Booz and Co.

United Nations (2013). *World population ageing 2013.* New York, United Nations (http://www.un.org/en/development/desa/population/publications/pdf/ageing/WorldPopulationAgeing2013.pdf, accessed 10 March 2016).

United Nations (2014). *World urbanization prospects, the 2014 revision.* New York, United Nations (http://esa.un.org/unpd/wup/highlights/wup2014-highlights.pdf, accessed 10 March 2016).

United Nations (2015). *World population prospects, the 2015 revision.* New York, United Nations (http://esa.un.org/unpd/wpp/publications/files/key_findings_wpp_2015.pdf, accessed 10 March 2016).

US-China Economic and Security Review Commission (2014). *2014 Report to Congress of the US-China Economic and Security Review Commission.* Washington DC, US-China Economic and Security Review Commission (http://www.uscc.gov/Annual_Reports/2014-annual-report-congress, accessed 10 March 2016).

US FDA (2013). *How many people are employed by FDA and in what areas do they work?* Washington, DC, US Food and Drug Administration (http://www.fda.gov/AboutFDA/Transparency/Basics/ucm213161.htm, accessed 10 March 2016).

Van Arnum P (2013). Evaluating China's supply chain: increased pharmaceutical trade creates new challenges for regulatory oversight. *Pharmaceutical Technology*, August, s30–s36.

Ventola CL (2010). Current issues regarding complementary and alternative medicine (CAM) in the United States. Part 2: regulatory and safety concerns and proposed governmental policy changes with respect to dietary supplements. *P T*, 35(9):514–522.

Vickers AJ, Cronin AM, Maschino AC, Lewith G, MacPherson H, Foster NE et al. for the Acupuncture Trialists' Collaboration (2012). Acupuncture for chronic pain: individual patient data meta-analysis. *Archives of Internal Medicine*, 172(19):1444–1453.

Vincent DW (2014). *Quality and compliance in the Asian pharmaceutical industry.* Burlington, MA, IVT Network (http://www.ivtnetwork.com/article/quality-and-compliance-asian-pharmaceutical-industry, accessed 10 March 2016).

Wagstaff A, Yip W, Lindelow M, Hsiao WC (2009). China's health system and its reform: a review of recent studies. *Health Economics*, 18(Suppl 2), S7–S23.

Wang C, Rao K, Wu S, Liu Q (2013). Health care in china improvement, challenges, and reform. *Chest*, 143(2):524–531.

Wang H, Zhai F (2013). Programme and policy options for preventing obesity in China. *Obesity Reviews*, 14:134–140.

Wang JH, Chen TY, Tsai CJ (2012). In search of an innovative state: the development of the biopharmaceutical industry in Taiwan, South Korea and China. *Development and Change*, 43(2):481–503.

Wang J, Wang P, Wang X, Zheng Y, Xiao Y (2014). Use and prescription of antibiotics in primary health care settings in China. *Journal of the American Medical Association Internal Medicine*, 174(12):1914–1920.

Wang K, Lin G (2014). Pharmaceutical IP and competition law in China: overview. *Practical Law*, May 1 (http://uk.practicallaw.com/0-568-3025, accessed 7 March 2016).

Wang L, Kong L, Wu F, Bai Y, Burton R (2005). Preventing chronic diseases in China. *Lancet*, 366(9499):1821–1824.

Wang W, McGreevey WP, Fu C, Zhan S, Luan R, Chen W et al. (2009). Type 2 diabetes mellitus in China: a preventable economic burden. *American Journal of Managed Care*, 15(9):593–601.

Wang W, Lau Y, Loo A, Chow A, Thompson DR (2014). Medication adherence and its associated factors among Chinese community-dwelling older adults with hypertension. *Heart and Lung*, 43(4):278–283.

Wang X, Fang Y, Yang S, Jiang M, Yan K, Wu L et al. (2014a). Access to paediatric essential medicines: a survey of prices, availability, affordability and price components in Shaanxi province, China. *PLOS ONE*, 9(3), e90365.

Wang X, He X, Zheng A, Ji X (2014b). The effects of China's new cooperative medical scheme on accessibility and affordability of healthcare services: an empirical research in Liaoning Province. *BMC Health Services Research*, 14(1):388.

Wang Y (2015). *NHPFC, MOF, State Council joint evaluation of public hospital reform.* Beijing, National Health and Family Planning Commission (http://www.cbda.cn/html/MDnews/20150729/64734.html, accessed 10 March 2016; in Chinese).

Wang Y, Li X, Zhou M, Luo S, Liang J, Liddell CA et al. (2015). Under-5 mortality in 2851 Chinese counties, 1996–2012: a subnational assessment of achieving MDG 4 goals in China. *Lancet*, 6736(15):1–11.

Wang YR (2006). Price competition in the Chinese pharmaceutical market. *International Journal of Health Care Finance and Economics*, 6:119–129.

Ward A (2014). GSK to pay £297m fine for Chinese bribes. *Financial Times* (http://www.ft.com/intl/cms/s/0/dea9811e-3fd5-11e4-936b-00144feabdc0.html#axzz3XNlPdfCs, accessed 10 March 2016).

WHO (2001). *How to develop and implement a national drug policy*, 2nd edn. Geneva, World Health Organization.

WHO (2014a). *China: noncommunicable diseases country profiles 2014*. Geneva, World Health Organization (http://www.who.int/nmh/countries/chn_en.pdf?ua=1, accessed 10 March 2016).

WHO (2014b). *Tobacco health warnings in China*. Geneva, World Health Organization.

WHO (2014c). WHO global health expenditure database [online/offline database]. Geneva, World Health Organization (http://apps.who.int/nha/database/ViewData/Indicators/en, accessed 10 March 2016).

WHO (2015a). Global Health Observatory data repository [online/offline database]. Geneva, World Health Organization (http://apps.who.int/gho/data/node.main.A867?lang=en, accessed 10 March 2016).

WHO (2015b). *Tobacco in China*. Geneva, World Health Organization (www.wpro.who.int/china/mediacentre/factsheets/tobacco/en/, accessed 10 March 2016).

WHO, Health Action International (2008). *Measuring medicine prices, availability, affordability and price components*, 2nd edn (http://www.who.int/medicines/areas/access/OMS_Medicine_prices.pdf, accessed 10 March 2016).

WHO, China National Health Development Research Center (2012). *Health service delivery profile: China*. Beijing, World Health Organization Country Office (www.wpro.who.int/health_services/service_delivery_profile_china.pdf, accessed 10 March 2016).

Withrow D, Alter DA (2011). The economic burden of obesity worldwide: a systematic review of the direct costs of obesity. *Obesity Reviews*, 12(2):131–141.

Woodhead M (2014). Hospitals sell off pharmacies to pharma companies. *China Medical News*, March 8 (http://www.chinesemedicalnews.com/2014/03/hospitals-sell-off-pharmacies-to-pharma.html, accessed 10 March 2016).

World Bank (2010). *Financing, pricing, and utilization of pharmaceuticals in China: the road to reform*. Washington DC, World Bank.

World Bank (2011). *Toward a healthy and harmonious life in China: stemming the rising tide of non-communicable diseases*. Washington DC, World Bank.

World Bank, State Environmental Protection Administration (2007). *Cost of pollution in China: economic estimates of physical damages*. Washington DC, World Bank (http://siteresources.worldbank.org/INTEAPREGTOPENVIRONMENT/Resources/China_Cost_of_Pollution.pdf, accessed 10 March 2016).

World Population Review (2016). *Major cities in China: population* (http://worldpopulationreview.com/countries/china-population/major-cities-in-china/, accessed 10 March 2016).

Wu B, Zhang Q, Qiao X (2014). Effects of pharmaceutical price regulation: China's evidence between 1997 and 2008. *Journal of the Asia Pacific Economy*, 20(2):290–329.

Wu J, Xu J, Liu G, Wu J (2014). Pharmaceutical pricing: an empirical study of market competition in Chinese hospitals. *PharmacoEconomics*, 32:293–303.

Wu Q (2015). *Precision medicine to be encouraged by 13th five year plan.* (http://finance.china.com.cn/industry/medicine/yyyw/20151029/3408884.shtml, accessed 10 March 2016; in Chinese).

Wu W-Y, Hou J-J, Long H-L, Yang W-Z, Liang J, Guo D-A (2014). TCM-based new drug discovery and development in China. *Chinese Journal of Natural Medicines*, 12(4):241–250.

Wu W-Y, Yang W-Z, Hou J-J, Guo D-A (2015). Current status and future perspective in the globalization of traditional Chinese medicines. *World Journal of Traditional Chinese Medicine*, 1(1):1–4.

Xiang X, Yang C, Wang D, Ye J, Zhang X (2012). Effects of China's national essential medicines policy on the use of injection in primary health facilities. *Journal of Huazhong University of Science and Technology, Medical Science*, 32(4):626–629.

Xiao Y, Li L (2015). The actions of China in containing antimicrobial resistance. *AMR Control*, 46–53 (http://www.globalhealthdynamics.co.uk/wp-content/uploads/2015/05/07_Xiao-Li.pdf, accessed 10 March 2016).

Xiao Y, Zhang J, Zheng B, Zhao L, Li S, Li L (2013). Changes in Chinese policies to promote the rational use of antibiotics. *PLOS Medicine*, 10(11):1–4.

Xin C, Xia Z, Jiang C, Lin M, Li G (2015). Effect of pharmaceutical care on medication adherence of patients newly prescribed insulin therapy: a randomized controlled study. *Patient Preference and Adherence*, 797.

Xu J, Yang Y (2009). Traditional Chinese medicine in the Chinese health care system. *Health Policy*, 90(2-3):133–139.

Xu Q, Bauer R, Hendry BM, Fan T-P, Zhao Z, Duez P et al. (2013). The quest for modernisation of traditional Chinese medicine. *BMC Complementary and Alternative Medicine*, 13:132.

Xue K (2015). *Li Keqiang announce major diseases scheme. Who benefits? Who will pay? How will it be implemented?* (http://info.pharmacy.hc360.com/2015/07/270910566332.shtml, accessed 10 March 2016; in Chinese).

Yan J (2013). *An overview: new drug registration system and approval process in China.* Beijing, Covance Pharmaceutical.

Yang C, Lei L (2010). Drug procurement bidding. *China Business Review,* January 1 (http://www.chinabusinessreview.com/drug-procurement-bidding/, accessed 10 March 2016).

Yang H, Dib HH, Zhu M, Qi G, Zhang X (2010). Prices, availability and affordability of essential medicines in rural areas of Hubei Province, China. *Health Policy and Planning*, 25(3):219–229.

Yang L, Sung H-Y, Mao Z, Hu T, Rao K (2011). Economic costs attributable to smoking in China: update and an 8-year comparison, 2000–2008. *Tobacco Control*, 20(4):266–272.

Yang L, Liu C, Ferrier JA, Zhou W, Zhang X (2012). The impact of the national essential medicines policy on prescribing behaviours in primary care facilities in Hubei province of China. *Health Policy and Planning*, 28(7):750–760.

Yang W, Lu J, Weng J, Jia W, Ji L, Xiao J et al. (2010). Prevalence of diabetes among men and women in China. *New England Journal of Medicine*, 362(12): 1090–1101.

Yang Z (2014). Kangmei pharmaceutical foray into drugstore trusteeship. *China Economic Net*, March 7 (http://en.ce.cn/Insight/201403/07/t20140307_2438194.shtml, accessed 10 March 2016).

Yao Q, Liu C, Ferrier JA, Liu Z, Sun J (2015). Urban–rural inequality regarding drug prescriptions in primary care facilities: a pre–post comparison of the national essential medicines scheme of China. *International Journal for Equity in Health*, 14(1):58.

Yao X, Wu J, Liu LL, Ye WW, Xue HBH, Montgomery W (2013). Medication use patterns and adherence after initiating antipsychotics treatment for patients with schizophrenia in Tianjin, China. *Value in Health*, 16(7), A554.

Yezli S, Li H (2012). Antibiotic resistance amongst healthcare-associated pathogens in China. *International Journal of Antimicrobial Agents*, 40(5):389–397.

Yi H, Miller G, Zhang L, Li S, Rozelle S (2015). Intended and unintended consequences of China's zero markup drug policy. *Health Affairs*, 34(8):1391–1398.

Yi Z-M, Zhao R-S, Zhai S-D, Yang L, Hu Y-F, Yang Y-H et al. (2014). Comparison of US and Chinese pharmacy education programs. *American Journal of Health-System Pharmacy*, 71(5):425–429.

Yip W, Eggleston K (2004). Addressing government and market failures with payment incentives: hospital reimbursement reform in Hainan, China. *Social Science and Medicine*, 58(2):267–277.

Yip W, Hsiao W (2014). Harnessing the privatisation of China's fragmented health-care delivery. *Lancet*, 384(9945):805–818.

Yip W, Powell-Jackson T, Chen W, Hu M, Fe E, Hu M et al. (2014). Capitation combined with pay-for-performance improves antibiotic prescribing practices in rural China. *Health Affairs*, 33(3):502–510.

Yip WCM, Hsiao WC, Chen W, Hu S, Ma J, Maynard A (2012). Early appraisal of China's huge and complex health-care reforms. *Lancet*, 379(9818):833–842.

Yi-Xin H, Manderson L (2005). The social and economic context and determinants of schistosomiasis japonica. *Acta Tropica*, 96(2–3):223–231.

Yoongthong W, Hu S, Whitty JA, Wibulpolprasert S, Sukantho K, Thienthawee W et al. (2012). National drug policies to local formulary decisions in Thailand, China, and Australia: drug listing changes and opportunities. *Value in Health*, 15:126–131.

Yu M, Zhao G, Stålsby Lundborg C, Zhu Y, Zhao Q et al. (2014). Knowledge, attitudes, and practices of parents in rural China on the use of antibiotics in children: a cross-sectional study. *BMC Infectious Diseases*, 14(1):112.

Yu X, Li C, Shi Y, Yu M (2010). Pharmaceutical supply chain in China: current issues and implications for health system reform. *Health Policy*, 97(1):8–15.

Yu Z, Han S, Chu J, Xu Z, Zhu C, Guo X (2012). Trends in overweight and obesity among children and adolescents in China from 1981 to 2010: a meta-analysis. *PLOS ONE*, 7(12), e51949.

Yusuf S, Saich T (2008). *China urbanizes: consequences, strategies, and policies.* Washington, DC, World Bank.

Zeng W (2013). A price and use comparison of generic versus originator cardiovascular medicines: a hospital study in Chongqing, China. *BMC Health Services Research*, 13(390):1–8.

Zhang D, Unschuld PU (2008). China's barefoot doctor: past, present, and future. *Lancet*, 372(9653):1865–1867.

Zhang F, Cooke PN, Wu F (2011). State-sponsored research and development: a case study of China's biotechnology. *Regional Studies*, 45:575–595.

Zhang F, Xie J-M, Zhang Y-Y, Kong L-L, Li S-C (2013). What is important during the selection of traditional Chinese medicine (TCM) in a health care reimbursement or insurance system? Critical issues of assessment from the perspective of TCM practitioners. *Value in Health Regional Issues*, 2(1):141–146.

Zhang H (2010). China's irrational medical pricing scheme. *Lancet*, 375(9716):726.

Zhang H-X, Li X, Huo H-Q, Liang P, Zhang J-P, Ge W-H (2014). Pharmacist interventions for prophylactic antibiotic use in urological inpatients undergoing clean or clean-contaminated operations in a Chinese hospital. *PLOS ONE*, 9(2), e88971.

Zhang J (2012). Comparing China's and India's pharmaceutical manufacturing. *Pharmaceutical Online*, August 30 (http://www.pharmaceuticalonline.com/doc/comparing-china-s-and-india-s-pharmaceutical-manufacturing-0001, accessed 10 March 2016).

Zhang J, Mauzerall DL, Zhu T, Liang S, Ezzati M, Remais JV (2010). Environmental health in China: progress towards clean air and safe water. *Lancet*, 375(9720):1110–1119.

Zhang J, Shi X, Liang X (2013). [Economic costs of both overweight and obesity among Chinese urban and rural residents, in 2010.] *Chinese Journal of Epidemiology*, 34(6):598–600.

Zhang L, Yan J, Liu X, Ye Z, Yang X, Meyboom R et al. (2012). Pharmacovigilance practice and risk control of traditional chinese medicine drugs in China: current status and future perspective. *Journal of Ethnopharmacology*, 140(3):519–525.

Zhang Q-Q, Ying G-G, Pan C-G, Liu Y-S, Zhao J-L (2015). Comprehensive evaluation of antibiotics emission and fate in the river basins of China: source analysis, multimedia modeling, and linkage to bacterial resistance. *Environmental Science and Technology*, 49(11):6772–6782.

Zhang S, Zhang W, Zhou H, Xu H, Qu Z, Guo M et al. (2015). How China's new health reform influences village doctors' income structure: evidence from a qualitative study in six counties in China. *Human Resources for Health*, 13(1):1–11.

Zhang X, Xiong Y, Ye J, Deng Z, Zhang X (2013). Analysis of government investment in primary healthcare institutions to promote equity during the three-year health reform program in China. *BMC Health Services Research*, 13(1):114.

Zhang X, Wu Q, Liu G, Li Y, Gao L, Guo B et al. (2014). The effect of the national essential medicines policy on health expenditures and service delivery in Chinese township health centres: evidence from a longitudinal study. *British Medical Journal Open*, 4(12), e006471–e006471.

Zhang Y, Ting RZ, Yang W, Jia W, Li W, Ji L et al. (2015). Depression in Chinese patients with type 2 diabetes: associations with hyperglycemia, hypoglycemia, and poor treatment adherence. *Journal of Diabetes*, 7(6):800–808.

Zhang YP, Deng MM (2008). Enforcing pharmaceutical and biotech patent rights in China. *Nature Biotechnology*, 26(11):1235–1240.

Zhao K (2014). *HTA in development assistance to health: potential and challenge in China*. Beijing, National Health Development Research Center.

Zhou M, Wang H, Zhu J, Chen W, Wang L, Liu S et al. (2015). Cause-specific mortality for 240 causes in China during 1990–2013: a systematic subnational analysis for the Global Burden of Disease Study 2013. *Lancet*, 6736(15):1–22.

Zhou Y, Lan-Juan L (2013). New medical reform and the sustainable development of the pharmaceutical industry in China. *Chinese Medical Journal*, 126(4): 775–782.

Zhou Z, Su Y, Campbell B, Zhou Z, Gao J, Yu Q et al. (2015a). The financial impact of the "Zero-Markup Policy for Essential Drugs" on patients in county hospitals in western rural China. *PLOS ONE*, 10(3), e0121630.

Zhou Z, Su Y, Campbell B, Zhou Z, Gao J, Yu Q et al. (2015b). The impact of China's Zero-Markup Drug Policy on county hospital revenue and government subsidy levels. *Journal of Asian Public Policy*, 8(1):102–116.

Zhou Z, Xue Y, Ping Q (2013). Consumer choice of purchasing private-label drugs: an empirical study in China. *Health Marketing Quarterly*, 30(4):349–361.

Appendix 1: Organizations participating in joint seminars

306th Hospital of the People's Liberation Army

Chinese Development Research Center of the State Council

Chinese Ministry of Human Resources and Social Security and provincial representatives

Chinese National Development and Reform Commission and provincial representatives

Chinese National Health and Family Planning Commission and provincial representatives

Chinese State Council Health Reform Office

Organisation of Economic Co-operation and Development

Peking Union Medical College

Peking University

Shanghai Medical Innovation and Development Foundation

Teda International Cardiovascular Hospital

World Health Organization China Office

World Health Organization Essential Medicines and Health Products Department

Various international academic institutions

Various international and domestic pharmaceutical companies

Appendix 2: Search terms for review of academic literature

The search was limited to English language academic papers published between 2005 and 2015.

MEDLINE

China and pharmaceutical policy

China and drug policy

China and medic* policy

China and pharma* and policy

China and drug* and policy

China and (drug* or medic* or pharma*) and reimbur*

China and (drug* or medic* or pharma*) and pric*

China and (drug* or medic* or pharma*) and generic*

China and (drug* or medic* pharma*) and irration*

China and (drug* or medic* pharma*) and prescrib*

China and (drug* or medic* pharma*) and (tender* or procure*)

Econlit

China and (drug* or pharma* or medic*) and policy

China and (drug* or pharma* or medic*) and reimbur*

China and (drug* or pharma* or medic*) and pric*

China and (drug* or pharma*) and generic*

China and (drug* or pharma*) and irration*

China and (drug* or pharma*) and prescrib*

China and (drug* or medic* pharma*) and (tender* or procure*)

Business Source Premier

China and (drug* or pharma* or medic*) and policy

China and (drug* or pharma* or medic*) and reimbur*

China and (drug* or medic* or pharma*) and pric*

China and (drug* or medic* or pharma*) and generic*

China and (drug* or medic* or pharma*) and irration*

China and (drug* or medic* pharma*) and prescrib*

China and (drug* or medic* pharma*) and (tender* or procure*)